FEARLESS
BEAUTIES

Treating Skin of Color with Confidence

SECOND EDITION

FEARLESS BEAUTIES

Treating Skin of Color with Confidence

MARY NIELSEN

EDITED BY
Jason Thomas

SECOND EDITION

SKINTELLIGENT RESOURCES • PORTLAND, OREGON

Skintelligent Resources.

Copyright © 2020 by Mary Nielsen.

All rights reserved. No part of this book may be used or reproduced in any form by an electronic or mechanical means (including photocopying or recording) without written permission from the publisher.

Printed in the United States of America.

Second Edition

Editor: Jason Thomas

Diversity Reader: Indu Guzman

Cover Design and Interior Layout by Sarah Jensen.

Cover Image by © Nadya_Art - Shutterstock.com.

ISBN 10: 0-9893-3456-3

ISBN 13: 978-0-9893-3456-3

18 19 20 21 22   CS   10 9 8 7 6 5 4 3 2 1

DEDICATED TO

Dedicated to the Fearless Beauties who are elevating our industry by being inclusive of all races, ethnicities, genders and cultures by acknowledging beauty exists in many forms and deserves honor and respect.

Why Fearless Beauties? AN INTRODUCTION	**01**
Asian Skin CHAPTER 1	**09**
Black Skin CHAPTER 2	**25**
South Asian Skin CHAPTER 3	**45**
Indigenous Skin CHAPTER 4	**65**
Latinx Skin CHAPTER 5	**83**
Nordic Skin CHAPTER 6	**99**
Multi-Ethnic Skin CHAPTER 7	**113**
Transgender Clients CHAPTER 8	**127**
Cultural Appropriation CHAPTER 9	**143**
Skin Classification Systems CHAPTER 10	**149**
Appendix A COMMON FORMS	**159**
Appendix B GLOSSARY	**183**

WHY FEARLESS BEAUTIES?

Fearless Beauties was born at this particular time and place in United States history because of a variety of intersecting societal, personal, and political events, which I'll cover in this intro. However, let's start off with the sentiment that drives me every day: it's time for a change in our aesthetics industry.

The mission of *Fearless Beauties* is this:

- To change the aesthetic education in our country by developing curricula that are inclusive of all ethnic, racial, and cultural backgrounds.
- To highlight entrepreneurs of color, on social media and at events, in order to increase their visibility and share their insights into success in the aesthetic industry.
- To become an influencer, so that our presence moves the needle toward equality in the field of aesthetics.

Graduates from cosmetology and aesthetics schools who are people of color (hereafter referred to as BIPOC) have no better education on treating their own skin than a white graduate of European heritage. Until now, aesthetic education catered to Western ideals of beauty, being fair-skinned, by teaching students how to care for Fitzpatrick skin types 1-3, while neglecting darker tones 4-6. Discussion on treating skin of color is still too often summed up in a few sentences that state skin of color is more challenging to treat and therefore requires additional classes to learn about. Information about ethnic skin is missing in standardized aesthetic textbooks but may be located in separate 'other' books that are not carried as part of a common curricula. Many school owners don't even know that these 'other' books exist because they are not readily available.

Our country is quickly transitioning to a multi-ethnic identity. In fact, the US population will be majority multi-ethnic within the next fifty years[1], meaning a country with a population of 'Blasian' (Black+Asian), 'Koreitalian' (Korean + Italian), and 'Vietino' (Vietnamese + Latino) is already in existence. *The Wall Street Journal* notes that in 2009, 3.5 million children were born and noted as being of two or more races on their birth certificates.[2]

The American cultural view of beauty is heavily Eurocentric, meaning it originated from European cultures that colonized North America in the late 1700s and 1800s. This Eurocentric approach came to America specifically from British domination, and as British rule exerted itself in each of its conquered countries, it demanded the Indigenous populations conform to European standards of dress, grooming, education, and social culture. Native traditions were frowned upon, swept aside, or, in some circumstances, completely lost.

Founded from these Eurocentric beginnings, white skin, blonde hair, and blue eyes are often considered the prized images of beauty today. Consumer marketing has reinforced these standards unapologetically through television, movies, magazines, and all forms of social media. Consider this case study: *Sports Illustrated* published its first Swimsuit Issue in 1964; the first model of color for this issue was featured on the cover in 1996–32 years later! In order to minimize any backlash from racist subscribers, the cover also featured a blonde-haired white model alongside the Black model, Tyra Banks (fig i.1). While I believe America is moving in the right direction by broadening the beauty standard to be more inclusive, we still have a long way to go.

The modern-day history of foundation makeup is another interesting case study on beauty. Using makeup for foundation began when Max Factor, a beautician from Poland, developed a line of pressed powder called Pan-Cake to even the skin tones of movie actors and actresses in the 1930s. The powder was meant to create a more natural finish as opposed to the heavy, greasy coverage derived from the greasepaint stage makeup of theatre.

As the 1940s ushered in World War II, women's beauty regimens were affected in order to support the war effort. Nylons, commonly produced as women's stockings, were now being used to create parachutes, rope, and rubber supplements. Women were encouraged to abandon their nylon stockings, even holding nylon drives at their local hosiery departments. Hence, "leg film" was born. This liquid foundation was marketed as a way to smooth and even out the appearance of white women's legs. It came in six shades and eventually evolved into liquid tinted bases for the face by the end of the 1940s (fig i.2).

Light shades of foundation makeup prevailed for decades while multimillion-dollar cosmetic companies largely ignored multi-ethnic populations by offering limited foundation colors. It wasn't until 2017 when Robyn Fenty, otherwise known as

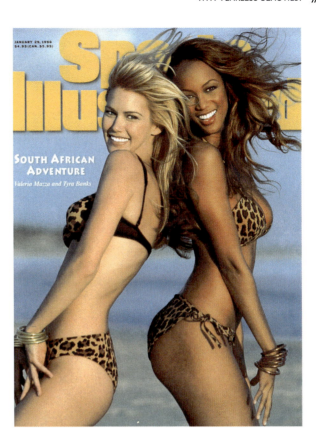

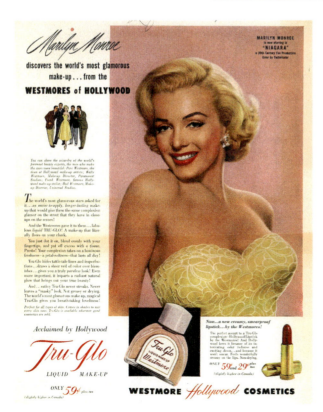

Top Image
Tyra Banks with Valerie Mazza on an iconic cover for the *Sports Illustrated* swimsuit edition. Photo source: *Sports Illustrated*, Cover.
(i.1)

Bottom Image
Marilyn Monroe, spokeswoman for TruGlo six shades of foundation. Photo source: *Life*, advertisement, Duke Digital Repository.
(i.2)

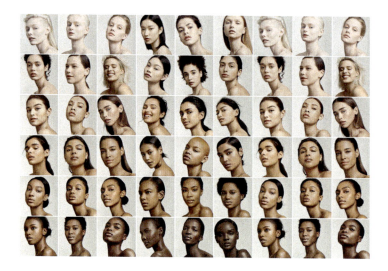

Rihanna opened the door to an untapped market with Fenty Beauty. Photo source: Fenty Beauty by Rihanna, "Thank you."
(i.3)

international pop star, Rihanna, caused a stir in the makeup world by releasing her cosmetic line, Fenty, with forty different shade options (fig i.3). Fenty's immediate success was a wakeup call to the beauty industry, proving that inclusivity in cosmetics is not just ethical but profitable.

Our country's current political climate, including the ascendancy of the 'Me Too' movement and the 'Black Lives Matter' movement, has highlighted the equality gap that still exists today. American beauty curricula have marginalized entire populations of our society by ignoring them, considering them as less-than, or pushing them to embrace Eurocentric beauty ideals. The aesthetics industry can do better. By developing aesthetic education that provides accurate, effective, and representative information on caring for skin of color, we are not just broadening education, we are doing the right thing.

On a personal level, I was awakened to the need for *Fearless Beauties* just a few short years ago. My youngest daughter was accepted by a small liberal arts college in Southern California called Occidental College. I was very proud of her decision to leave a small, blue-collar, mostly white town and open her world view by moving to Los Angeles, one of the most diverse cities in our country. Her classes were intentionally filled with students from a variety of racial, ethnic, and cultural backgrounds, and I was impressed with how my daughter began thinking of others' experiences as she moved through the world on her own. One day she made the statement, "Not everyone sees the world through the same lens that you do." Those words were an epiphany to me.

I wish that I was aware of differences earlier in my career and I wish I had encouraged more inclusivity in esthetics education earlier in founding my esthetics school. But because of my Viking heritage, I am committed to being fierce and unafraid of change. I am fully Scandinavian and grew up in a small town in Minnesota. Although the entire town's population had Nordic features of blue eyes, blonde hair, and fair skin, the inhabitants had their own cultural biases against each other. I clearly remember my father telling me, 'You're a Norwegian and don't let anyone call you a Swede.'

I want this industry that I love and that has given me such fulfillment to be awakened to the need for education that addresses inclusivity and equality for all. It is professional progression, but more than that, it's personal. These days I'm a part of a blended family with two of my four children marrying partners who are BIPOC. Some of my grandchildren are multi-ethnic. This is a trend that is based not solely on my experience but is reflected in advertising, television programming and Hollywood films.

The claim that 'everyone is beautiful' is professed loudly and frequently by cosmetic brands, however it should be validated by making services, treatments, and products available to all ethnic, cultural, and racial backgrounds. As Americans, we need to recognize and legitimize that minorities within our country may have different standards for beauty and different ways of honoring and respecting that beauty. By developing a more inclusive education, we elevate our entire industry.

Furthermore, *Fearless Beauties* has a vision to highlight the success of minority entrepreneurs in order to increase their visibility within our industry. We celebrate all achievements in order to inspire our community of skincare professionals and elevate all of us into more profitable and meaningful careers.

Notes

1. William H. Frey, "The US will become 'minority white' in 2045, Census projects," *Brookings*, March 14, 2018, https://www.brookings.edu/blog/the-avenue/2018/03/14/the-us-will-become-minority-white-in-2045-census-projects/.

2. Gretchen Livingston, "The rise of multiracial and multiethnic babies in the U.S.," *Pew Research Center*, June 6, 2017, https://www.pewresearch.org/fact-tank/2017/06/06/the-rise-of-multiracial-and-multiethnic-babies-in-the-u-s/.

Fig i.1. "South African Adventure Valeria Mazza and Tyra Banks," *Sports Illustrated*, January 29, 1996, cover.

Fig i.2. "Marilyn Monroe Discovers The World's Most Glamorous Make-up...From The Westmores of Hollywood," *Life*, 1952, advertisement, Duke Digital Repository, https://idn.duke.edu/ark:/87924/r4h41k76j

Fig i.3. Fenty Beauty By Rihanna (@fentybeauty), "Thank you to the 1 Million #fentyfamily that agree that beauty is inclusive of all," Instagram photo, September 12, 2017, https://www.instagram.com/p/BY9PocNlkFm/?utm_source=ig_embed.

1

ASIAN SKIN

ASIAN SKIN

Beatrice is a 35-year-old Vietnamese-American woman (fig 1.1). She looks younger than her age and walks with confidence and purpose. Beatrice was born in the United States after her parents immigrated here with the fall of Saigon in the late 1970's, seeking economic opportunity and escaping a country in chaos (fig 1.2).

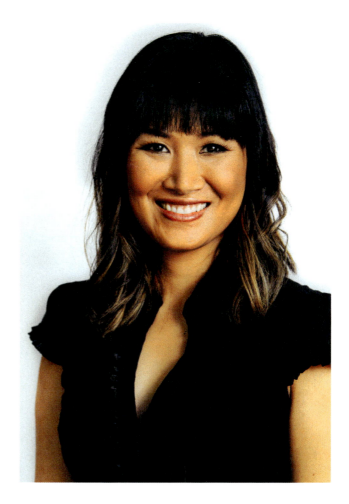

Beatrice, Dermascope's 2018 Favorite Esthetics Educator. Photo source: Megan Rayo, Electric Beauty Productions.
(1.1)

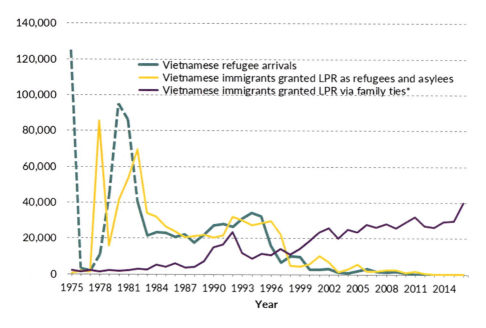

Vietnamese Refugee Arrivals and Vietnamese Immigrants Granted Lawful Permanent Residence (LPR) as Refugees and Asylees or through Family Ties, 1975-2016. Graph source: Alperin and Batalova, "Vietnamese Immigrants," fig.7.
(1.2)

Beatrice's childhood memories include working at her parent's deli. Clearing and setting tables as a child progressed to different duties at the deli, she worked through high school and even college where she majored in biology. The deli is where she developed her multi-tasking capabilities, people skills, budgeting, and time management. Bea is a Type A personality with a competitive desire to be at the top of her game. She challenges herself to stay physically fit, researches nutrition and health, and takes time to nurture her marriage and her personal relationships.

While in college, a part-time job at the front desk of a new Medi-Spa introduced Beatrice to aesthetics. She was hooked. She completed her aesthetics training and began working in medical aesthetics, performing laser hair removal and skin rejuvenation treatments when laser aesthetics was still in its infancy. Technology hadn't advanced to the stage where treating Asian skin could be performed safely.

What Are the Characteristics

Thankfully technology has progressed and science has been established that identifies the unique characteristics of Asian skin.

- Asian skin is thinner.
- Despite thinner skin, Asian skin has the benefits of a thicker dermis, so Asian skin is more resistant to aging (fig 1.3). More melanin in the basal layer helps protect against premature aging from sun damage.
- Asian skin has greater trans-epidermal water loss (TEWL) than other ethnicities.
- Asian skin is more sensitive to environmental factors. The pH balance is more easily disrupted, which leads to barrier function issues.
- Asian skin typically has fewer hair follicles but larger eccrine glands. This can make pores seem larger.
- Larger eccrine glands mean oilier skin, so Asian skin often battles acne. Even without acne, Asian skin deals with unwanted shine (fig 1.4).

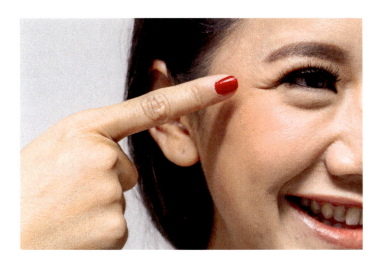

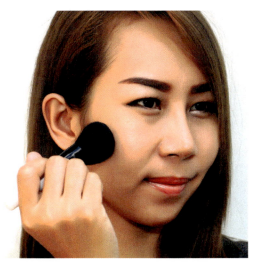

Top Image
Asian skin is more resistant to aging.
Photo source: twinsterphoto/123rf.com.
(1.3)

Bottom Image
Asian skin deals with unwanted shine.
Photo source: Sumetee Theesungnern/123rf.com.
(1.4)

Diseases and Disorders

There are a few diseases and disorders that Asian skin encounters more frequently than other ethnicities with Fitzpatrick skin types 1 through 3.

- Post-inflammatory hyperpigmentation or PIH is significant. Any injury to the skin, including a tiny disruption to the epidermis, can cause melanocytes to overproduce. Dark red lesions form in areas where an assault to the skin has occurred, oftentimes inflammation due to an acne breakout assault. It's important for the new aesthetician to identify post-inflammatory hyperpigmentation as an inflammatory condition rather than active acne. The dark red spot may be visible as a sign that an acneic lesion was present but it is now in the healing phase. Because the skin is more sensitive, be careful not to over treat with drying agents or harsh ingredients.

- Acne is another common disorder that afflicts Asian skin because of the larger eccrine glands. A build-up of sebum, debris and dead skin cells can block the pore and can create comedones, pustules, and even cystic lesions under the skin (fig 1.5). Acne studies show that acne sufferers are not able to produce enough of an enzyme that breaks down the debris in the follicle. The follicle becomes plugged and this warm, moist environment is the perfect breeding ground for the *p.acnes* bacteria.

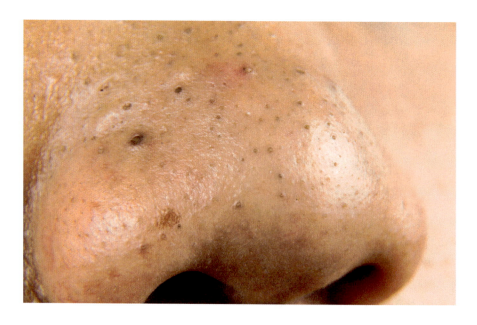

A close up of blackheads on a nose caused when pores are clogged with oil, dead skin cells, and/or bacteria. Photo source: thamkc/123rf.com.
(1.5)

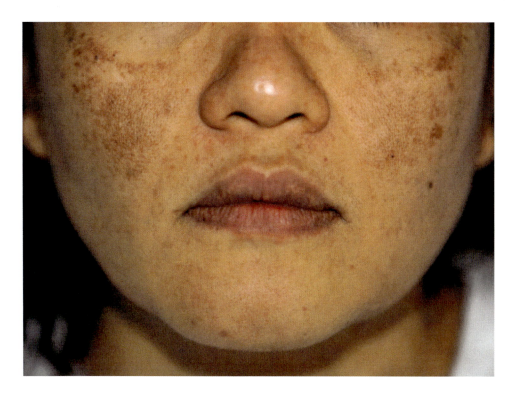

Symmetrical patches of dark melasma discoloration present on the cheeks of an Asian woman. Photo source: Oats.chumnak/Shutterstock.com.
(1.6)

- Asian skin is susceptible to melasma. Melasma is a hyperpigmentation disorder, often associated with a hormonal imbalance, that causes diffuse and dark pigmentation that is typically symmetrical on both the right and left sides of the face (fig 1.6). It can often have a 'butterfly' appearance across the cheeks and nose. It is also evident on the forehead, chin, and upper lip. It can appear during pregnancy or with the start of oral contraceptives. It is thought that there may be a genetic component. Thyroid disorders and phototoxic reactions to certain medications can also bring out melasma. Once those melanocytes have been triggered to overproduce, it is virtually impossible to turn them off. Most skin care professionals will use a combination or variety of treatments and skin care products to keep the hyperpigmentation under control.

- Seventy-five to one-hundred percent of Chinese, Korean and Japanese people have a genetic inability to digest lactose.[1] In addition to the symptoms of bloating, excess gas, and diarrhea, lactose intolerance can cause skin rash, hives and inflammation. Symptoms of eczema can be eliminated or reduced with the elimination of dairy from the diet.

- Atopic dermatitis is a condition that affects Asian skin because of its higher trans-epidermal water loss or TEWL (fig 1.7). This affects the skin's barrier function and create irritation with ingredients that have fragrances, or high concentrations of alpha hydroxyl or salicylic acids. When you are working with Asian clients, be cautious about recommending a skin care regimen with too many active ingredients. Even long chain peptides can cause irritation. Introduce products gradually and build in strength as your client's skin becomes conditioned.

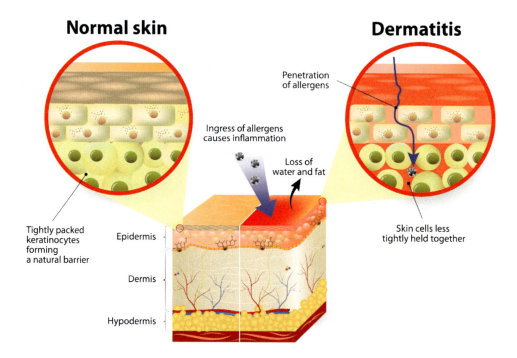

Diagram showing differences between skin afflicted with atopic dermatitis and normal skin. Photo source: designua/123rf.com.
(1.7)

Cultural and Dietary Practices

During consultation, investigate deeper into the cultural practices your Asian client may be observing. This will help you identify skin disorders and better educate your client on healthy skin practices.

Asian culture is not homogeneous but made up of many cultures with distinct languages and practices. The US census identifies more than 25 distinct Asian ethnic groups. The cultural and dietary practices discussed in this book are intended as generalizations and not specific to one particular client or ethnic group.

Many Asian cultures use traditional medicine and treatments that may produce unfamiliar effects on the body. Coin-rubbing, for instance, is a practice where a coin is rubbed on the body in an effort to remove toxins, eliminate diseases, and return the body to a state of homeostasis and more energy.[2] The effects from coin rubbing can appear like bruises on your client's body (fig 1.8).

Ingestion of herbal supplements, particularly ginseng, is taken to help reduce stress. Ingesting large amounts of ginseng can also cause a tendency to bruise and bleed.

Many spices used in Asian dishes, like turmeric, cumin, ginger, and lemongrass, have anti-inflammatory properties.

Many Asian-Americans do not use sunscreen because they are under the misconception that they have enough melanin to protect their skin from the negative effects of UV radiation in sunlight. Asian skin does have more melanin

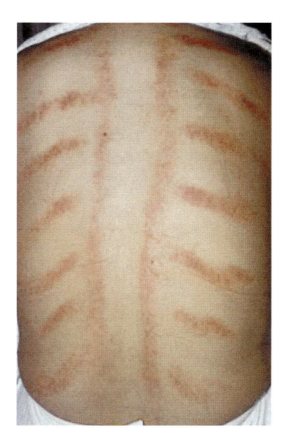

Ecchymosis produced by coin-rubbing (Gua sha), a technique often used in traditional East Asian medicine. Photo source: Jin, Slomka, and Blixen, " Cultural and clinical issues," 56, fig.1.
(1.8)

protection as it has the classification of a Fitzpatrick skin type 4. Your client will tan easily, rarely burn, and have dark hair and eyes.

Most Asian cultures value lighter skin and clients will often incorporate herbal skincare remedies to lighten pigmentation. Before French colonialism in Vietnam instilled the Eurocentric ideation of white skin being more beautiful, Asian social status was already defined by skin color. A person with darker skin had a lower social status because darker skin often indicated this person worked outdoors in a manual labor job and thus had a lower economic position. A person with lighter skin was assumed to have a higher social status because that person was not exposed to the elements of working outside and may have had an inside office job or other position with a greater economic stature.

The Consultation

A consultation with your Asian client will set the stage for a successful treatment plan. Your consultation needs to dive into your client's medical history as well as their skin care regimen, cultural practices, and diet, and a physical examination of the skin (fig 1.9).

Your intake form should include a question asking your client what ethnicity they identify with and a Fitzpatrick skin type identification. Your client may have skin that looks like a Fitzpatrick 2–light skin, eyes, and hair–but also have characteristics unique to Asian skin.

Asian skincare routines can be very intense. Korean routines, in particular, incorporate a ten or more step process (fig 1.10).

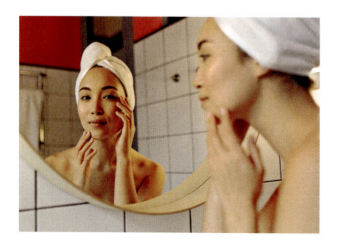

Learning about a client's home skincare routine is an important part of the consultation. Photo source: Look Studio/Shutterstock.com.

(1.9)

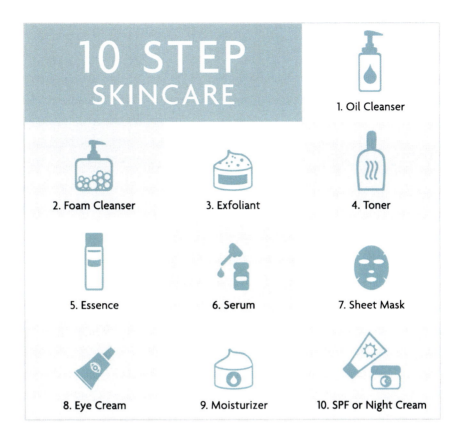

Typical Korean ten step skincare regimen. Graphic source: magic pictures/Shutterstock.com, edited by Sarah Jensen.
(1.10)

Being knowledgeable about the routine will help you in your skin analysis. Is your client's skin naturally dry or is it dehydrated? Is the skin inflamed or sensitive? Is your client exfoliating too frequently? Is the serum too harsh? A good grasp on ingredients and their actions will elevate your professional credibility.

Ask your client questions about their diet. Are they unknowingly contributing to inflammation in their skin by ingesting dairy? Are they eating a diet rich in omega fatty acids, healthy fats, and antioxidants to maintain a strong barrier function and reduce trans-epidermal water loss? Is your client well hydrated? What about their caffeine intake? Are they losing hydration from the diuretic effects of caffeine?

Carefully examine your client's skin after cleansing. Look under magnification and observe pore size, texture, and tone. Note pigmentation and look for melasma. A thorough examination will include checking elasticity, redness and inflammation, as well as telangiectasias, evidence of post-inflammatory hyperpigmentation, and active acne.

Get photos of your client's skin as a baseline for comparison. Get photos in a front view and side views.

The consultation is not a quick five minute process. You are becoming familiar with your client's skin and making determinations for a treatment plan that should include professional treatments and home skincare recommendations. Ask for clarifications on what your client has completed on the intake form to ensure you are gaining a strong comprehension of the unique characteristics of their skin. Make notes to refer to later and take your time. You are developing a relationship with your client, and the time you take in the beginning will help reduce or eliminate potential problems in the future.

The Treatment Plan

The consultation will give you the information to formulate a treatment plan that will include professional skincare sessions as well as home skincare recommendations. You are not 'selling' to your client, but using your professional expertise to educate your client on the best options for returning their skin to health.

Professional treatments should be started progressively. You will have to condition your client's skin to prevent adverse reactions. Explain to your client that you are offering a treatment plan that will condition their skin to gradually reach results and reduce the risk of PIH and atopic dermatitis because you understand the complexities of their Asian skin.

Microdermabrasion/Infused Microdermabrasion

Asian skin can tolerate mild microdermabrasion treatments. An aggressive treatment can disrupt barrier function, increase inflammation, and compromise TEWL. Build your client's skin tolerance by increasing the aggressiveness of the treatments when done in a series. Give your client's skin time to heal between sessions.

Chemical Peels

Asian skin can respond well to chemical peels. You are going to condition your client's skin response and build their tolerance. When the product is applied, your client should never feel that the discomfort level is above a 5 on a scale of 1 to 10.

The peel may not ever give your client visible sheets of skin peeling from the skin, but will cause a micro-shedding exfoliation.

If your client has never experienced professional skincare treatments before, start with a mild enzyme peel. When your client can tolerate an enzyme peel you can progress to a gentle alpha hydroxy acid peel. Malic acid, mandelic acid, and mid-pH, low-percentage glycolic acid peels are excellent options. In a series of peels, increase the strength over a period of months.

Facial Devices

Facial devices are a great option for creating healthy skin with your Asian client. Devices like microcurrent, ultrasonic and galvanic iontophoresis can make significant changes in Asian skin. Just remember to use your device with a progressive rather than aggressive approach. A series of treatments will build your client's tolerance and increase their skin conditioning, similar to the way going to the gym can increase your body's strength.

Lasers and IPL

Your Asian client may respond well to laser and IPL treatments for pigmentation, fine lines, texture, and pore size. You should never use an IPL to treat melasma. The laser or IPL device must be FDA registered to treat darker Fitzpatrick skin types. You should never exceed the manufacturer's suggested parameters for treatment. Always treat progressively rather an aggressively.

LED light therapy is a treatment that will enhance the effects of other treatments and will relieve inflammation and erythema.

Combination Treatments

Your clients will benefit from combination treatments that approach skin problems from different angles. Alternating treatment modalities with the tools in your aesthetic toolbox, such as fractional laser sessions, mild chemical peels, radio frequency, microneedling session, and mechanical exfoliation will strengthen your client's ability to tolerate more aggressive treatments and reach your client's skincare goals.

Pretreating your client's skin with skincare that inhibits melanin production before beginning a series of treatments, and continuing your client on melanin inhibitors will reduce the risk of hyperpigmentation. You will have to balance your recommendations of skin lighteners that cause irritation with moisturizers that have calming and soothing properties.

Home Skincare Recommendations

Explain to your client that you are offering a treatment plan that will condition their skin to gradually reach their skin care goals and that you have training in the best ways to treat Asian skin. This will help your client have confidence in your abilities.

Home care should include a gentle cleanser and pH balancing toner. Caution your client against exfoliating too frequently. Begin with single-ingredient serums. Combination serums may be too aggressive and may cause irritation and inflammation. As your client develops a tolerance and their skin becomes more conditioned, you can incorporate stronger serums.

If your client is seeing you for hyperpigmentation issues, it's best to start them on a melanocyte inhibitor that is plant-fungus-based. This will condition their skin to accept a low-dose hydroquinone product for a short-term therapeutic session. Hydroquinone is a controversial skincare ingredient but it has a place in treating challenging pigmentation for short-term use. Transition them from 2% hydroquinone to a 4% hydroquinone and then back to a plant based melanocyte inhibitor over a course of six to eight months. Your client should see pigmentation begin to blend, but during times of hot weather, they may have to increase their topical application or titrate in some topical hydroquinone for a short time again.

Your client may need a light moisturizer to keep lipids balanced. A moisturizer that is too heavy may increase risk of acne breakouts due to eccrine gland secretions.

You will need to educate your client on the importance of SPF and reinforce the need for UV protection.

If your client is being treated for acne, you will use the same progressive rather than aggressive approach. Common ingredients that are effective against acne, such as benzoyl peroxide, salicylic acid, and other alpha hydroxy acids can be effective at thinning the stratum corneum and keeping the follicle open but you will have to condition your client's skin gradually. Starting too aggressively will dehydrate your client's skin and possibly compromise barrier function.

Conclusion

Asian skin has its own distinctive needs, and a skilled and educated professional can provide an effective skincare treatment plan and make recommendations for home skincare. The patience to move your client in a progressive series of treatments will lower the risk of adverse reactions. Increasing client loyalty and elevating your profession are the results of knowing the unique characters of your client's skin.

NOTES

1. G. Flatz and Ch. Saengudom, "Lactose Tolerance in Asians: a Family Study," *Nature* 224 (Nov 1969): 915-916, https://doi.org/10.1038/224915a0.

2. Xian Wen Jin, Jacquelyn Slomka, and Carol E. Blixen, "Cultural and clinical issues in the care of Asian patients," *Cleveland Clinic Journal of Medicine* 69, no. 1 (Jan 2002): 56-57.

Fig 1.2. Elijah Alperin and Jeanne Batalova, "Vietnamese Immigrants in the United States," Migration Policy Institute, September 13, 2018, fig 7, https://www.migrationpolicy.org/article/vietnamese-immigrants-united-states-5

Fig 1.8. Xian Wen Jin, Jacquelyn Slomka, and Carol E. Blixen, "Cultural and clinical issues in the care of Asian patients," *Cleveland Clinic Journal of Medicine* 69, no. 1 (Jan 2002): 56, fig. 1.

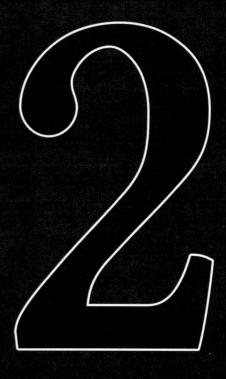

2

BLACK SKIN

BLACK SKIN

Amber is a fierce advocate for changing our American ideal of beauty. She grew up in southern California and Portland, Oregon where her family strived to find a middle-class living (fig 2.1). She attended Oregon State University after high school, majoring in anthropology. She has an easy smile and friendly eyes, and her full hair is a striking attribute that she takes pride in.

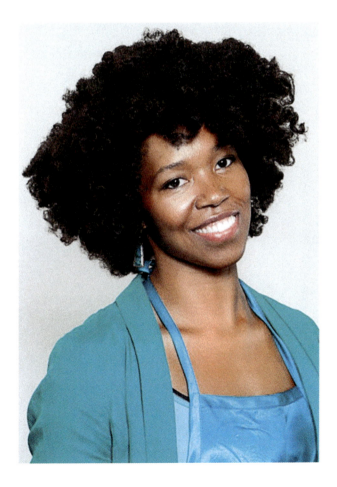

Amber Starks of Conscious Coils in Portland, Oregon. Photo source: Amber Starks.
(2.1)

Amber has become an advocate for natural beauty. She hosted a TED Talk about embracing the beauty of her African features. She spoke of wanting a blonde hair, blue eyed doll as a child because she never saw dolls with skin her color. Our culture does not represent diversity well, especially in the beauty business. After years of attempting and failing to tame her hair into submission, she finally embraced it and opened a natural hair care salon in Portland, Oregon. She works in the cultural tradition of hair braiding and was instrumental in bringing natural hair care licensing to Oregon.

Meet Wairimu (fig 2.2). Wairimu's mother embraced Wairimu's father's Kenyan origins and started a West African dance troupe and an African drumming group, while Wairimu was growing up in Eugene, Oregon. Her mother researched and incorporated Kenyan music and other cultural influences into their family life.

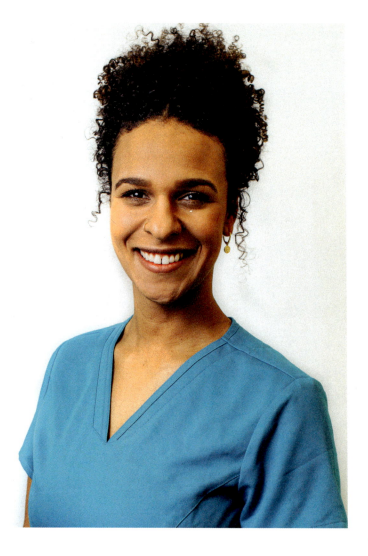

Wairimu, Advanced Esthetician.
Photo source: Megan Rayo, Electric Beauty Productions.
(2.2)

In Kenya, the social culture is group-oriented rather than individualistic. The country's motto is "Harambee" meaning "to pull together." It is a concept that identifies the population's belief in mutual effort, mutual responsibility, and helping your fellow man.[1]

Eugene is a mid-size city in Oregon and home of the University of Oregon (Go Ducks!) but lacks diversity. Only 1.4% of the population is Black, while 86% of the population is white.[2] Despite the lack of diversity, Wairimu never noticed her skin color was darker than her friends until the 4th grade. During a dance class, while picking out costumes, she suddenly became aware of how her skin looked different from her classmates. In high school, she went through a phase of wanting to look more like her friends with blonde straight hair because our culture was emphasizing the looks of Britney Spears and other white beauty icons. She didn't have examples of ethnic beauty to validate her own looks.

Wairimu began her journey to aesthetics during high school when she began styling her friends' hair and makeup for dances, proms, and other events. After finishing high school, she entered cosmetology school, intending on getting a license in hair design. She eventually shifted to an aesthetics course of study, as the science and technology involved in treating skin became more interesting to her. She still does her friends' hair, but it's more of an artistic outlet as aesthetics is her career of choice.

What Are the Characteristics

Black skin has its own unique characteristics. These include the following:

- More layers of keratinized cells in the stratum corneum.
- Larger sebaceous glands are evident in Black skin.
- Greater transepidermal water loss (TEWL), creating skin that is more sensitive, despite larger oil glands.
- Melanosomes have larger granules with a deeper disbursement in the basal layer of the epidermis.
- More melanin and, therefore, greater UV protection resulting in the skin aging more slowly (fig 2.3).
- Facial muscles display less movement, so there is a reduced tendency to develop signs of aging, such as creases between the brows and crow's feet.

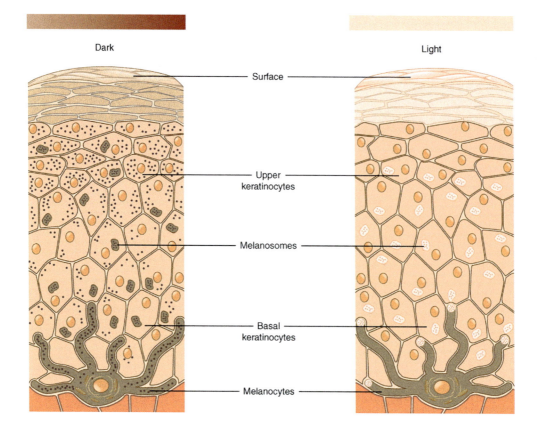

Diagram showing skin pigmentation. The relative coloration of the skin depends on the amount of melanin produced by melanocytes in the stratum basale and taken up by keratinocytes. Diagram source: Betts et al., *Anatomy and Physiology*, 188, figure 5.8.
(2.3)

Diseases and Disorders

- Post-inflammatory hyperpigmentation (PIH) is the largest concern for darker Fitzpatrick skin types. Any irritation to the skin can result in dark, purplish lesions that can take months to fade or never fade.

- Melasma is a challenge in Black skin because many treatments to correct melasma involve creating an inflammatory response, which could result in PIH. Melasma can be evident on the skin due to hormonal imbalances, as well as some prescription medications. There is a hereditary component to melasma, but it is not well understood.

- Dermatosis papulosa nigra is a hyperpigmentation disorder characterized by multiple small brown to black papules on the face (fig 2.4). They are not cancerous but can become a cosmetic concern if they grow in size.

- Pseudofolliculitis barbae is a challenging issue for Black men and some Black women. The hair follicle is curved and the hair curls back into the skin. These ingrown hairs can cause keloid scarring and PIH.
- Keloid scarring is an overgrowth of scar tissue after an injury (fig 2.5). The tissue that grows to repair the injury stays within the confines of the original scar but becomes elevated and thick.
- Hypertrophic scarring is similar to keloid scarring, but the scar tissue extends beyond the borders of the original scar.

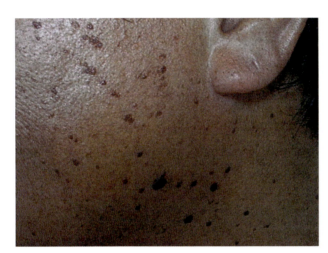

Top Image
Dark colored papules of dermatosis papulosa nigra on the cheek. Photo source: Duffill, "Dermatosis," DermNet NZ.
(2.4)

Bottom Image
A keloid scar. Photo source: Weerachat Chatroopamai/123rf.com.
(2.5)

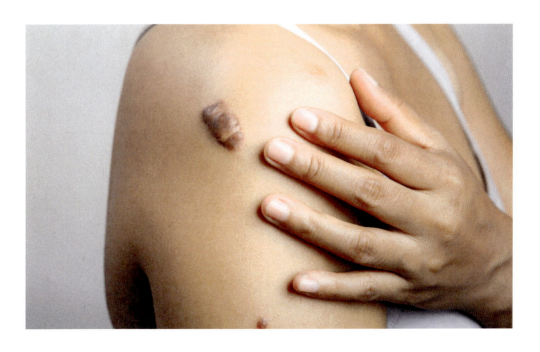

- Polycystic Ovarian Syndrome (PCOS) is a significant issue for Black women (fig 2.6). The symptoms of PCOS include acne and hirsutism. Women with PCOS have metabolic issues with weight gain, as well as insulin resistance, difficulty regulating blood sugar, and male-pattern hair loss.

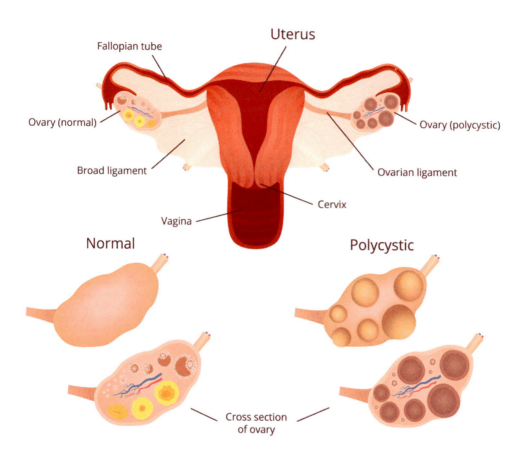

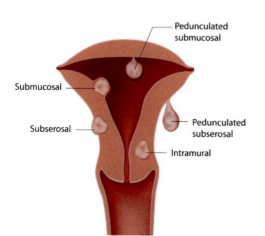

Top Image
Normal uterus and ovaries vs polycystic ovarian syndrome. Illustration source: Anasnasiia Lavrenteva/123rf.com.
(2.6)

Left Image
Five different types of uterine fibroids. Illustration source: alila/123rf.com.
(2.7)

Right Image
Bristol Stool Chart. Chart source: Sarah Jensen.
(2.8)

- Uterine fibroids are three times more common in Black women than in white women. Uterine fibroids are non-cancerous growths in the uterine wall that grow singly or in clusters (fig 2.7). Twenty-five percent of young Black women, 50% of middle aged Black women, and 80% of older Black women suffer from uterine fibroids. Some research indicates that it could be related to genetics, obesity, diet, the age that the woman had her first menstrual cycle, and the use of hair relaxers. Studies done in 2009 indicate that there is an association between the onset of menstruation and the use of hair relaxers. This may be a factor in Black women beginning menstruation earlier than women of other ethnicities.

- Constipation is an issue, especially when combined with uterine fibroids. In fact, one of the symptoms of uterine fibroids is constipation. Black women may not even be aware that constipation is significant. Bowel movement frequency is not a topic that is discussed in detail in any situation, even medical evaluations. Women who have a bowel movement weekly, bi-weekly, or monthly may assume their bowel habits are normal.[3] The Bristol Stool Chart was designed by two physicians in Great Britain in 1997 in order to facilitate medical consultations (fig 2.8).

1		Separate hard lumps, like nuts	Severe constipation
2		Lumpy and sausage like	Mild constipation
3		A sausage shape with cracks in the surface	Normal
4		Like a smooth, soft sausage or snake	Normal
5		Soft blobs with clear-cut edges	Lacking fiber
6		Mushy consistency with ragged edges	Mild Diarrhea
7		Liquid consistency with no solid pieces	Severe Diarrhea

- Acne is common with Black skin because of its larger sebaceous glands and extra layers of stratum corneum that impede the shedding of keratinocytes. The follicle is blocked resulting in retention keratosis. The keratinized cells are trapped in the follicle, and thus dead cells and debris collect resulting in inflammation. Pustules follow with the growth of bacteria.

- Acne on the back, neck, chest and upper arms is often linked to constipation. Treating the constipation with probiotics and a high-fiber diet will help clear the acne.

- Vitamin D deficiency may be an issue with Black women of Muslim faith who wear burqas. The practitioner should be aware that burqas filter out UV rays, and women who wear them often suffer from vitamin D deficiencies, which can cause fatigue, hair loss, impaired healing, and bone loss.

Cultural and Dietary Practices

In the sixteenth century, Africa was a thriving and diverse continent with many developed nations with advanced cultures and philosophies. The introduction of the slave trade and colonialism in the eighteenth and nineteenth centuries caused a significant loss in culture and traditions that could be passed from one generation to the next. Cultural practices were often transferred by oral history. Family units were broken apart and geographically dispersed; in the Americas, African traditions were replaced and African-American traditions developed.

In recent history, Black beauty was ignored by mainstream society. This was acutely evident in our country's obsession with beauty pageants. The first beauty pageant was organized by P. T. Barnum in 1854. In 1921, over 100,000 people saw sixteen-year-old Margaret Gorman crowned the first Miss America, garnering her public acclaim and a $100 prize.

Black communities began hosting their own beauty pageants, acknowledging a different standard for beauty (fig 2.9). These standards still tended to favor lighter skin, and controversy still surrounds this ideal. Consumer marketing reinforces this ideal of lighter skin and dialogue continues as Black celebrities have their images photoshopped to have lighter skin. A high percentage of Black women use some type of skin lightener in their skin care routine. Statistics from 2017 report the skin lightening is a $4.8 billion dollar industry globally and is expected to double in growth by 2027.[4]

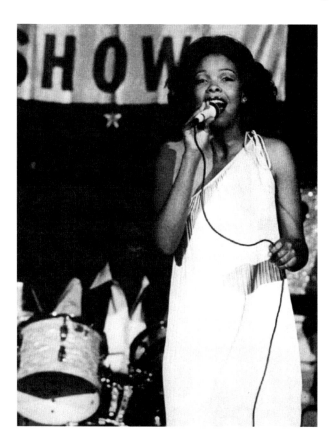

1977 Miss Black America winner, Claire Ford, performing during a United Service Organizations show, circa 1978. Photo source: Mitchell, "Miss Black America," 8.
(2.9)

Her win was in 1983, even though her title went into effect in 1984, Vanessa Williams became the first African-American woman crowned Miss America, sixty-three years after Margaret Gorman won her crown. She was criticized by some in the Black community for not being "Black enough" with her "coffee with creamer" skin, hair that was considered not "curly enough" and eyes that were considered not "dark enough."[5]

Howard University was the first college built exclusively for Black Americans. Howard University began organizing its own beauty pageant in 1939, focusing on entrants who embodied community service. Criteria was redefined and favored those who embraced the civil rights movement in the 1960s. To this day, the tradition is still strong and has added a Beauty King to the Beauty Queen coronation.[6]

Black women are divided in their hair care practices with most Black women (and men) practicing some form of hair straightening. Images of Black celebrities in the 1950s and 1960s, including Sammy Davis Jr., Nat King Cole, and Lena Horne all have straightened hair. African Americans adopting natural hair styles have emerged or re-emerged as a source of ethnic pride in recent history.

Black women with natural hair styles often wrap their hair in silk scarves at night. This information can be valuable when evaluating a client's acne, as acne around the hairline may be attributed to the head scarf.

One of the first Black female entrepreneurs in the United States was Sarah Breedlove, aka Madam C. J. Walker,[7] who recognized the monetary power behind the Black consumer (fig 2.10). Madam C. J. Walker preceded Oprah as the wealthiest Black women by founding a hair and skin care company that targeted Black consumers in 1906. She and her husband traveled the United States to educate Black communities on Black haircare and skincare. She even started a beauty school and founded her own manufacturing company (fig 2.11).

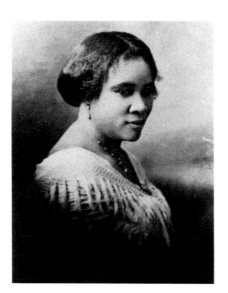

Top Image
In 1906 Madam C.J. Walker began marketing her own hair care line. Her success continued to grow and by 1911 the Madam C.J. Walker Manufacturing Company was incorporated. This photograph was used extensively in her advertisements and company literature. Not only was she an extremely successful business woman but she was also know for her work in social and civil rights activism as well as for her philanthropy. Photo source: Madam C.J. Walker Collection, Indiana Historical Society.
(2.10)

Bottom Image
A photograph of the product line at the Madam C.J. Walker Manufacturing Company. Products shown include: Wonder Pomade for Men, Vegetable Shampoo, Tan-Off, Vanishing Cream, Tetter Salve, Floral Cluster, and Grower. Photo source: Madam C.J. Walker Collection, Indiana Historical Society.
(2.11)

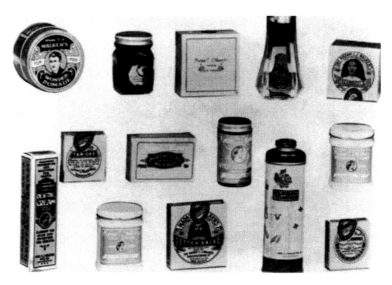

Black owned beauty salons have been places of community gathering and support.[8] The beauty salon offers a location where information is shared, values are enforced, and local gossip is rehashed. Political viewpoints are dissected. The salon becomes a secure place where social justice issues are discussed. This gathering place offers strength to the community to voice the need for changes in standards of beauty.[9]

There are some dietary traditions in the Black communities that are holdovers from the days of slavery.[10] Plantation owners would give their slaves the leftovers or what wasn't considered fit for white consumption. Often this included the internal organs of animals. The adoption of this food is regarded the origin of "soul food." Chitlins, animal intestines that are boiled and then fried, for instance, are a staple.

Studies indicate there is a higher percentage of Black Americans who are in a lower socioeconomic status and live without access to fresh produce. The food that is available often contains a lot of processed ingredients.[11] Black American children have higher obesity rates, in part, because of these factors. Since estrogen is stored in fat, this contributes to hormonal disorders.

The Consultation

You want to ensure you are allowing time for a thorough consultation with your client. Review your client's medical history. You're going to be getting personal, and you need to gain their trust. Giving the appointment your full attention will result in a better outcome for your client.

Be sure to discuss your client's tendency to scar, and look for keloids or hypertrophic scarring. Ask them about their tendency for hyperpigmentation. When it occurs, how long does it last?

Hyperpigmentation is the most common reason clients seek treatment so be sure to carefully determine whether your client has melasma or sun damage.

A solid skin analysis will help you determine your client's skin type: oily, dry, sensitive, or normal. Does your client have dry, flaky, dull-looking skin or do they battle shininess and congestion?

Zero in on their menstrual history, possibility of fibroids, or polycystic ovarian syndrome. You can't make a diagnosis, but if you suspect your client may have hirsutism or acne because of an endocrinological or reproductive disorder, refer them to a medical professional for evaluation. You can begin to treat the symptoms of the condition, but a sound medical diagnosis will help set the appropriate expectations for your clients.

Asking about your client's bowel habits may seem unusual, but you need to know your client's bowel regularity. The way you phrase your question, such as asking about "bowel habits" and not "pooping" will validate your professionalism. Explaining the relationship between bowel habits and acne could be helpful.

Ask your client about their medications. Are any photosensitizing?

Does your client wear a silk scarf at night? How often do they change it? It could be contributing to their hairline acne.

Is your client eating a diet of fresh vegetables and fruit with enough protein, or does their diet have a high level of processed food and not enough water?

Ask about your client's home care regimen. They may be using a topical lightener that could interfere with the home skincare treatment plan you recommend for them. They may resist discontinuing the lightener, so you'll have to find ways to work around it.

Does your client have specific goals? Do they have an event coming up or a special occasion that they are preparing for?

Verify your client's allergies. If you're going to be performing chemical peels, your client's allergies are important knowledge and will make a difference in the type of peel you select for your client.

Use the Fitzpatrick scale to get a generalized idea of your client's skin type in relation to UV exposure.

Before photos are important so you have a baseline for comparison. Get photos in multiple views.

The Treatment Plan

Your consultation will guide you to the best treatment plan for your client. Take some time to review all of the details you have acquired in the consultation before you forge ahead with developing the treatment plan.

Since pigmentation will be one of the biggest issues facing you and your client, you need to be confident in your approach to pigmentation. Any treatment plan will have to consider the repercussions from post-inflammatory hyperpigmentation (PIH).

Inform your client that changes to their skin will be a process and improvements will be incremental, since aggressive treatment will risk long-term PIH. They should appreciate your cautiousness and reassurance that you have their best interests in mind.

Instruct your client on a series of professional treatments as well as a home skincare regimen (fig 2.12).

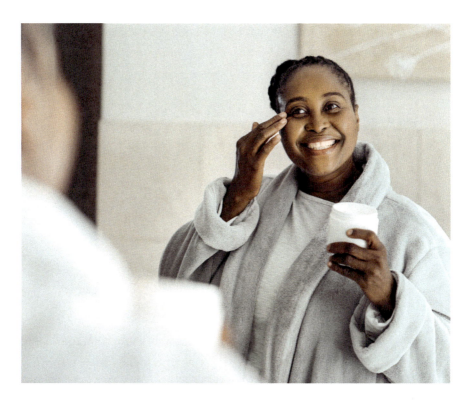

Professional treatments must be partnered with home skincare. Photo source: mavoimages/stock.adobe.com.
(2.12)

Microdermabrasion/Infused Microdermabrasion

Black skin can tolerate microdermabrasion if it is oily, dry, or combination skin. Sensitive skin should not receive microdermabrasion. Because of the risk of PIH, begin with a mild microdermabrasion or wet microdermabrasion for the first session. Removing the excess stratum corneum is a great approach to introducing home skincare, as well as introducing other professional treatments. Your acneic client should see some improvements in their breakouts even with the first treatment.

Chemical Peels

Black skin responds well to a series of chemical peels of increasing intensity. Do not start aggressively, so you aren't risking PIH as a side effect.

Glycolic acid is your strongest peel. It has the smallest molecule and will penetrate the deepest. Be mindful of which acids are hydrophilic and which acids are lipophilic.

The first peel should be an enzyme. If your client can tolerate an enzyme peel, the next peel in the series should be a low-percentage acid with a relatively high pH. You can alternate an AHA with a BHA. Your client may not have visible peeling. In fact, visible peeling may be too aggressive and could result in hyperpigmentation. Microscopic sloughing is your target.

Build your client's skin strength by increasing the percentage of acid or decreasing the pH slightly. With this approach you are exercising your client's skin and increasing your ability to be more aggressive with your treatments.

Facial Devices

Black skin may respond well to low-level facial devices. Ultrasonic spatula, high frequency, and galvanic are all add-on facial options that may bring improvements to your client's skin.

For more invasive treatments, do a skin test first to determine appropriateness. Take keloid scarring and hyperpigmentation in consideration when using treatments like microneedling. If you feel your client can tolerate microneedling, begin slowly with a shorter needle depth and fewer passes than you would with white skin.

Lasers and IPL

Fractional laser treatments are an option with Black skin when the skin is appropriately conditioned with a series of chemical peels and home skincare that includes a melanocyte suppressant.

1064 Nd: YAG is considered the gold standard for treating skin of color.

IPL is NOT a treatment modality for Black skin because of the concentration of melanocytes in the dermis and epidermis.

Though some companies will claim that their device is capable of safely treating Fitzpatrick skin types 5 and 6, you must remember that the intense pulsed light energy will be activated in the skin for hours after the treatment, and negative reactions may not be fully visible until the next day.

Radio frequency collagen induction therapy is gaining in popularity and could be an effective option for your client's skincare needs, but caution is needed, and including test pulses will make you confident in your approach toward treatment.

If you are using high-powered devices, you need to verify that the device is FDA approved for treating your client's Fitzpatrick skin type and never exceed the manufacturer's recommended guidelines for settings.

Combination Treatments

Your client can benefit from treatments that approach the skin differently. Alternating modalities will condition your client's skin and build the ability to use stronger acids or device settings; however, the skin must be pretreated with melanocyte inhibitors first to reduce the possibility for PIH. Balance your recommendations of skin lighteners containing irritating ingredients with moisturizers that have calming and soothing properties.

Your clients will benefit from combination treatments that approach the skin problem from different angles. Alternating treatment modalities with the tools in your aesthetic toolbox, such as fractional laser sessions, mild chemical peels, radio frequency, microneedling session, and mechanical exfoliation will strengthen your client's skin.

LED light therapy is a great combination therapy. Green light can help with pigmentation; red light is anti-aging; and blue light is effective for acne.

Home Skincare Recommendations

Your client may not have a lengthy history of professional skincare when they come to you, so you need to spend time explaining the importance of home care. Eighty percent of their results will come from the home care that is partnered with the professional treatments. Add products to their home care regimen one at a time, so if they have a problem, you can easily recognize which product is causing the irritation or inflammation. You can steadily add more potent ingredients as you become familiar with their skin's reactions and tolerance levels. Beware of harsh ingredients that compromise transepidermal water loss (TEWL), since it may result in rebound oiliness.

As you incorporate ingredients, start your client on a gentle cleanser and pH-balancing toner.

Although the use of hydroquinone is controversial, you can recommend short-term use to get pigmentation under control and reduce melanin production. Titrate your client from a 2% hydroquinone once a day for three weeks to twice a day for three weeks. Then increase the hydroquinone dosage to 4% in the morning, and continue with the 2% dosage in the evening for three weeks. Finally, increase the evening hydroquinone application to 4% so your client is using 4% hydroquinone twice daily for three weeks. By this time, the pigmentation should be noticeably improved. You can titrate your client off the hydroquinone and onto a non-hydroquinone melanocyte inhibitor. Your client may have times when they need to switch back to hydroquinone, such as during hot summer weather when melanin activity is very active.

Make your moisturizer recommendation based on your skin assessment. Your client may need lighter hydration if their skin is oily and heavier hydration if they have drier skin.

Introduce epidermal growth factors and antioxidant serums slowly to nourish the skin and build collagen. First, have your client use them twice a week for two weeks. Then, increase to three times a week for two weeks. After that, increase to every other day for two weeks. Finally, increase your client's regimen to daily use.

You may have to introduce sunscreen to your client. Inform them that people with Black skin are still at risk for skin cancer if sunscreen is not applied.

When working with an acneic client, avoid products that are harsh and drying as they can result in rebound oiliness and increased acne breakouts. Low-percentage salicylic acid usually works well due to its antimicrobial properties. Retinol is often sensitizing to Black skin, so use it cautiously.

Conclusion

You can treat your client with Black skin with confidence when you take a progressive rather than aggressive approach. Gain your client's trust with strong consultation skills, explaining that treating skin of color is a journey that involves gradual treatment and minimizing the risk of PIH.

Elevate your profession by being knowledgeable about all skin types. Black skin has specific needs, and you need to be skilled in treating a population that has been marginalized throughout history and largely ignored by the beauty industry.

NOTES

1. "Kenya - Language, Culture, Customs and Etiquette," Commisceo Global Consulting Ltd, accessed March 26, 2019, https://www.commisceo-global.com/resources/country-guides/kenya-guide.

2. "Eugene Population," World Population Review, December 27, 2018, accessed March 26, 2019, http://worldpopulationreview.com/us-cities/eugene-population/.

3. "Learn How to Treat Multicultural Skin," Joelle, accessed March 26, 2019, https://www.joelleskincare.com/esthetics-training.

4. Coco Khan, "Skin-lightening Creams Are Dangerous – Yet Business Is Booming. Can the Trade Be Stopped?," *The Guardian*, April 23, 2018, https://www.theguardian.com/world/2018/apr/23/skin-lightening-creams-are-dangerous-yet-business-is-booming-can-the-trade-be-stopped.

5. Annys Shin, "In 1983, Vanessa Williams Became the First Black Miss America," *The Washington Post*, September 14, 2017, https://www.washingtonpost.com/lifestyle/magazine/in-1983-vanessa-williams-became-the-first-black-miss-america/2017/09/11/9b99a4fe-81d0-11e7-ab27-1a21a8e006ab_story.html?utm_term=.5b86f9707d4e.

6. Jennifer C. Thomas, "Pageantry & Politics: Miss Howard University from Civil Rights to Black Power," *The Journal of Negro Education*, 87, no. 1 (2018): 22-32, https://www.jstor.org/stable/10.7709/jnegroeducation.87.issue-1.

7. Maxine Leeds Craig, "Black Women and Beauty Culture in 20th-Century America," *Oxford Research Encyclopedia of American History*, (November 2017), https://dx.doi.org/10.1093/acrefore/9780199329175.013.433

8. "The Community Roles of the Barber Shop and Beauty Salon," National Museum of African American History and Culture, accessed March 26, 2019, https://nmaahc.si.edu/blog/community-roles-barber-shop-and-beauty-salon.

9. Catherine Davenport, "Skin Deep: African American Women and the Building of Beauty Culture in South Carolina," (master's thesis, University of South Carolina, 2017), https://scholarcommons.sc.edu/etd/4201/

10. Jazz Keyes, "Slave Food: The Impact of Unhealthy Eating Habits on the Black Community," *EBONY*, March 29, 2017, accessed March 26, 2019, https://www.ebony.com/health/black-health-food-diet/.

11. Iris Mansour, "How Access to Fresh Food Divides Americans," *Fortune*, August 15, 2013, accessed March 26, 2019, http://fortune.com/2013/08/15/how-access-to-fresh-food-divides-americans/.

Fig 2.3. J. Gordon Betts et al., *Anatomy and Physiology* (Houston: OpenStax, 2013), chap. 5, 188, fig. 5.8, https://openstax.org/details/books/anatomy-and-physiology.

Fig 2.4. Mark Duffill, "Dermatosis papulosa nigra," DermNet NZ, 2008, https://www.dermnetnz.org/topics/dermatosis-papulosa-nigra/.
https://creativecommons.org/licenses/by-nc-nd/3.0/nz/legalcode

Fig 2.9. Terry Mitchell, "Miss Black America," U.S. Navy All Hands, May 1978, 8, https://www.navy.mil/ah_online/archpdf/ah197805.pdf
The appearance of U.S. Department of Defense (DoD) visual information does not imply or constitute DoD endorsement.

Fig 2.10. Addison Scurlock, Madam C.J. Walker, 1910s, Photograph, Madam C.J. Walker Collection, Indiana Historical Society, http://images.indianahistory.org/cdm/singleitem/collection/m0399/id/228/rec/13.

Fig 2.11. Madam C.J. Walker Product Line, Photograph, Madam C.J. Walker Collection, Indiana Historical Society, http://images.indianahistory.org/cdm/singleitem/collection/m0399/id/1920/rec/332.

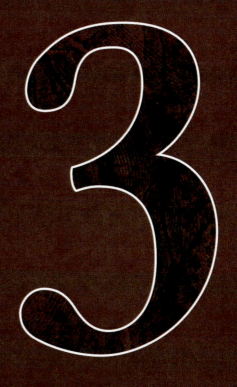

3

SOUTH ASIAN SKIN

SOUTH ASIAN SKIN

When we discuss South Asian skin, we are referencing people from Bhutan, India, Pakistan, Sri Lanka, Bhutan, The Maldives, Afghanistan, Nepal and Kashmiri. South Asia used to represent the south region of the Asian continent. It is bound by the Indian Ocean to the south and by West Asia, Central Asia and Southeast Asia.

Anna is a dynamic thirty-year-old woman who enjoys the outdoors (fig 3.1). An avid hiker, she sees beauty in nature.

Anna's beginnings were meager. She called an orphanage in India home for her first two years. Her mother, thousands of miles away in Oregon, had a vision that

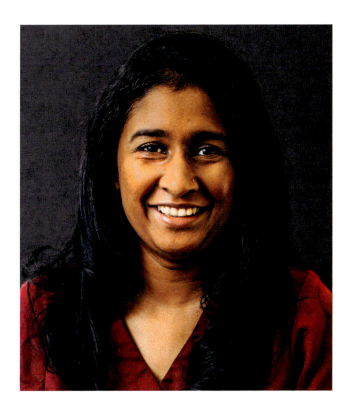

Anna, Esthetics Educator and Advanced Esthetician. Photo source: Megan Rayo, Electric Beauty Productions.

(3.1)

she should adopt a girl from India. Her husband didn't agree at first, but when he had a dream where Jesus was handing him a baby girl with dark skin, he became a believer. Their church rallied behind their vision and contributed money toward an adoption fund (fig 3.2).

She grew up in small town in southern Oregon, secure in the love of her family and free to run and play outside and use her imagination. She has a love of animals and a strong loyalty to family and friends. As a teenager, Anna was a skin product junkie struggling with acne, which led her mother to encourage her to seek a career in aesthetics after high school. She excelled at a prestigious East Coast aesthetic school and returned to the Pacific Northwest.

She worked close to ten years in dermatology offices, helping clients with acne and performing other treatments that improved a variety of skin conditions, as well as performing aesthetic treatments like laser hair removal. Her community had ethnic diversity with a Latinx population, but few of South Asian descent. She's had few resources to learn about her own skin type. She felt a calling to share her knowledge of medical aesthetics with students and currently works in an aesthetic school, encouraging and mentoring new skincare enthusiasts.

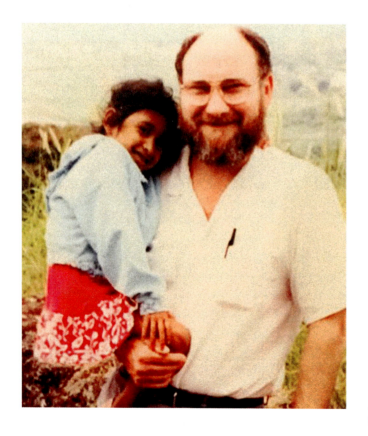

Anna and her father. Photo source: Anna L.
(3.2)

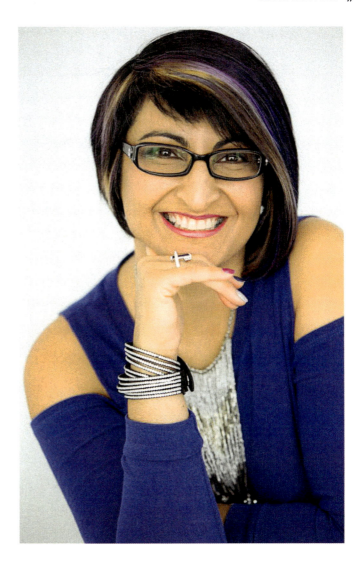

Tazeem, Esthetic Mentor and Spa Business Coach. Photo source: Tazeem Jamal.
(3.3)

Tazeem brings a forward-thinking global perspective to her aesthetics career (fig 3.3). She was born in Tanzania, Africa and was raised in London. Her private all-girls school and finishing school education paid off in dividends when she immigrated to British Columbia, Canada to begin her livelihood in aesthetics. Two years after being licensed, at age twenty, she ventured into her own practice, building her location from scratch. Success led to expansion and expansion led to building a custom spa with a focus on acquiring the affluent client. The universe met her expectations, and she was wildly successful until the economic downturn in 2008. She was forced to close her business and mourned its loss for two years before realizing that she could use her expertise of 25 years in the aesthetics business to coach new aestheticians to start their own businesses and achieve success.

What Are the Characteristics

Research from *National Geographic* has plotted the migration of early humans (fig 3.4). Prehistoric South Asians migrated mainly north through Mongolia, China and into North America. A smaller percentage of the South Asian population migrated south to Australia.[1]

- South Asian skin has many similarities to Western European skin. Oil gland and hair follicle distribution are congruent. The number of melanocytes is the same, but melanosome production is second only to Black skin.

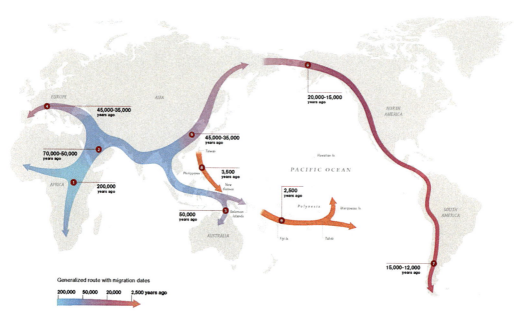

Generalized route of modern human migration out of African some 60,000 years ago. Map source: *National Geographic*, "Global Human Journey."
(3.4)

Diseases and Disorders

South Asian skin battles some issues that are similar to other Fitzpatrick skin types 4 through 6, but two are unique.

- Paradoxical hair growth is a unique characteristic of South Asian/Mediterranean skin. Paradoxical means contradictory. Treatment for hair removal may actually cause the rare side effect of fine hair growth instead.

It's a phenomenon that's not well understood, but studies indicate it most often happens with the 755 nm alexandrite wavelength. It typically occurs in areas where South Asian women have downy hair, usually the sides of the face, edges of the forehead, and back of the neck (fig 3.5). Instead of hair loss, women experience a denser hair growth pattern.

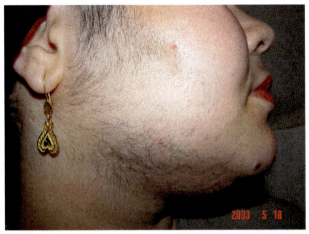
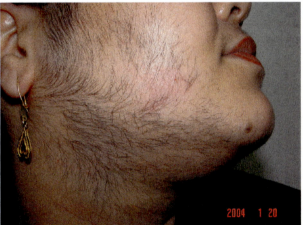

Paradoxical hair growth. Photo source: Radmanesh, "Paradoxical," 52-54, fig. 1 & fig. 2.
(3.5)

- Periorbital hyperpigmentation is another unique characteristic of South Asian and Mediterranean peoples. Periorbital means "around the eyes." Dark circles under and around the eyes is a condition that is not well understood. Numerous studies have been done by respected South Asian medical professionals, and it seems that a combination of factors contribute toward its severity. There is a genetic component as well as a hormonal component, since it seems to affect women more predominantly than men.

The skin around the eye is the thinnest on the body and supported with a fragile vascular system (fig 3.6). The leakage of tiny vessels increases the risk of hemosiderin staining. Red blood cells in the vessels returning blood to the heart become fragile and break down, leaving iron deposits. Often the pigmentation increases with age, due to thinning of the already thin skin around the eyes, exposure to UV, smoking, and diet.

The degree of hyperpigmentation is ranked on a scale from 1 to 4:

Grade 1 is faint pigmentation of the infraorbital area (fig 3.7).

Grade 2 has more pronounced pigmentation (fig 3.8).

Grade 3 has deep color and involves top and bottom eyelids (fig 3.9).

Grade 4 extends beyond the infraorbital fold (fig 3.10).

South Asian consumers spend an enormous amount of money on products attempting to improve dark circles around the eyes, but there doesn't seem to be an effective remedy to eliminate them. Hydroquinone products can provide some relief but can be very irritating to delicate eye tissue. Also, since ochronosis occurs more often in skin of color, hydroquinone may be a short term remedy, if alternated with other melanocyte or tyrosinase inhibiting eye creams. Combination therapy seems the most effective, although no options provide a permanent solution. We'll discuss possible treatment options in the Treatment Plan section of this chapter.

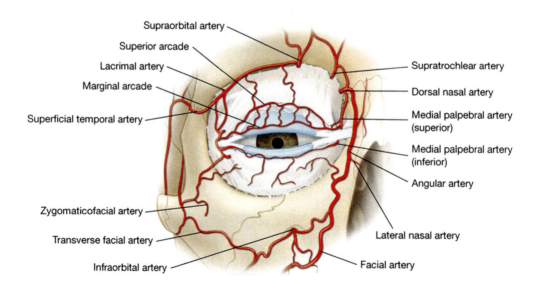

Periocular microvasculature. Photo source: Alghoul et al., "Eyelid Reconstruction," 288e-302e.

(3.6)

SOUTH ASIAN SKIN // 51

Periocular hyperpigmentation
Grade 1. Photo source: Sheth, Shah, and Dave, "Periorbital" 151-157, fig.5.
(3.7)

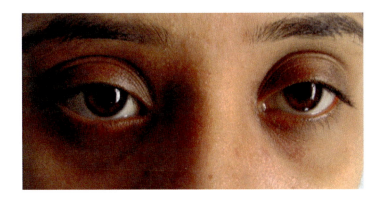

Periocular hyperpigmentation
Grade 2. Photo source: Sheth, Shah, and Dave, "Periorbital," 151-157, fig.1.
(3.8)

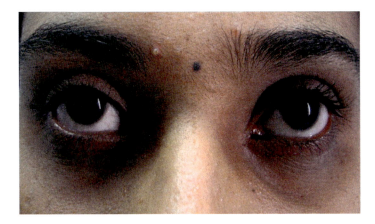

Periocular hyperpigmentation
Grade 3. Photo source: Sheth, Shah, and Dave, "Periorbital," 151-157, fig.6.
(3.9)

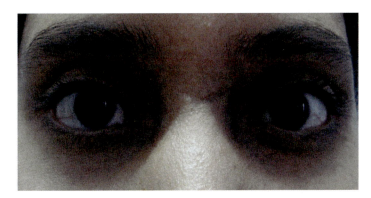

Periocular hyperpigmentation
Grade 4. Photo source: Sheth, Shah, and Dave, "Periorbital," 151-157, fig.7.
(3.10)

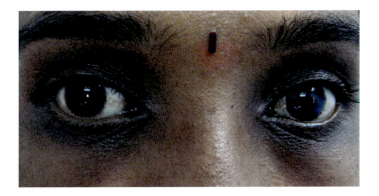

- South Asian skin will easily hyperpigment after an injury. Even insect bites can leave a long lasting mark. Post-inflammatory hyperpigmentation in South Asian skin will cause damage to the basal layer as basal keratinocytes leak melanin. Melanophages, macrophages filled with melanin, accumulate in the dermis, and dermal hyperpigmentation is created. In some cases, PIH can last years before fading.

- Acne is the fourth most common skin disorder within the South Asian population. It is believed that South Asian and Western European acne develops in the same way; the hair follicle becomes plugged due to the pilosebaceous unit's inability to shed the accumulating keratinocytes and sebum. One of the most challenging issues in treating acne with South Asian skin is managing the PIH that occurs with papules, pustules, and cysts.

- South Asian skin is also susceptible to melasma. Hyperpigmented brown to grayish brown macules appear in a symmetrical pattern on the face. Twenty to thirty percent of South Asian women ages forty to sixty-five have melasma. Researchers believe that genetic predisposition, increased estrogen levels, possible ovarian dysfunctions, thyroid dysfunctions, and liver dysfunctions, as well as exposure to UV radiation and some medications interact to stimulate the melanogenesis in melanoma.

- South Asian skin, among other darker Fitzpatrick skin types, can experience hyperpigmentation due to a Vitamin D deficiency.[2]

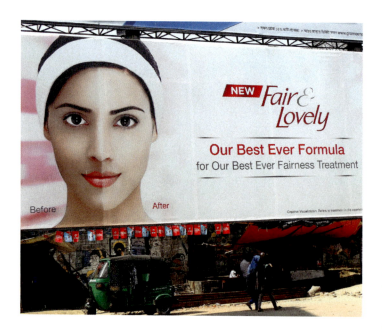

A billboard advertising Fair & Lovely skin whitening cream in Chittagong, Bangladesh.
Photo source: Jones, *Fair and Lovely*.
(3.11)

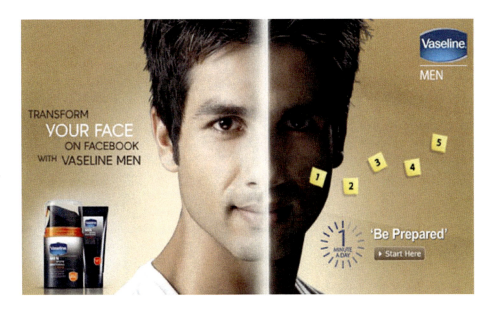

Skincare group Vaseline introduced a skin-lightening application for Facebook in 2010. It was designed to promote a growing line of skin-lightening creams for men. The app encouraged men to "Be Prepared" by whitening their profile pictures. Photo source: Whiteman, "Vaseline," CNN.
(3.12)

Cultural and Dietary Practices

South Asian culture is still influenced by "shadeism," which traces back to 100 BC. A caste social system valued light skin, promoting the message that light skin meant higher intelligence, worth, and privilege. Current South Asian beauty culture continues to value light skin. Consumer marketing is directed toward home lightening agents (fig 3.11).

Light skin is so valued that there is a phone app that will lighten skin in photos to post on social media (fig 3.12).

Current South Asian culture prizes Ayurvedic skincare products. Ayurvedic medicine, which originated in India more than 3000 years ago, is popular worldwide as a holistic practice of health. Ayurvedic medicine practitioners believe that a person's health is controlled by a delicate balance between the mind, body, and spirit. According to Ayurveda, every person is made of five elements: space, air, fire, water, and earth. The five elements combine and form three different life forces, or life energies, called *doshas*. Everyone has a unique *dosha* mix of space and air, or fire and water, or water and earth. Although everyone has all three *doshas*, one *dosha* is stronger than the others. Keeping the *doshas* balanced will affect a person's health.

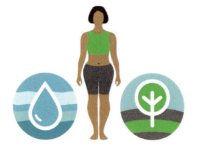

KAPHA

Qualities that reflect water and earth
heavy, stable, moist, smooth, oily, slow, sweet

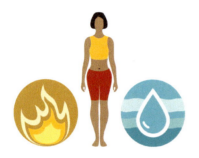

PITTA

Qualities that reflect fire and water
hot, sharp, slightly oily, liquid, sour, quick moving, pungent

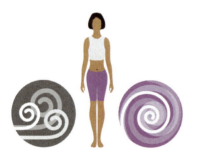

VATA

Qualities that reflect space and air
dry, light, moving, cold, rough, subtle, astringent, bitter

The Ayurvedic body types and their corresponding elements. Illustration source: voinsveta and Yana Alisovna/stock.adobe.com, edited by Sarah Jensen.
(3.13)

South Asians who practice Ayurvedic medicine believe in the Ayurvedic body types (fig 3.13). A Vata body type is lean with little muscle. A Pitta body type is well muscled, and a Kapha body type is stocky and stout.

Mehndi is a type of body adornment using henna, a paste made from the henna plant, used in religious ceremony, especially to adorn a bride for her engagement and wedding ceremony (fig 3.14). Indian wedding celebrations are multi-day events, and one day is solely dedicated to adorning the bride and the groom, known as 'Mehndi ki raat'.

Indian dishes are spiced with anti-inflammatory and antioxidant rich spices, including turmeric, curries, and peppers (fig 3.15).

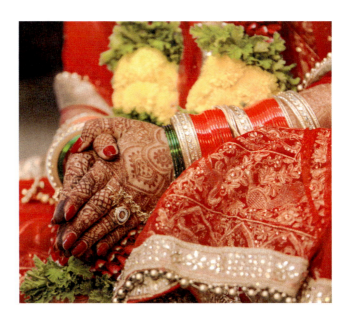

Traditional Mehndi on a bride's hand. Photo source: Ashish_wassup6730/Shutterstock.com.
(3.14)

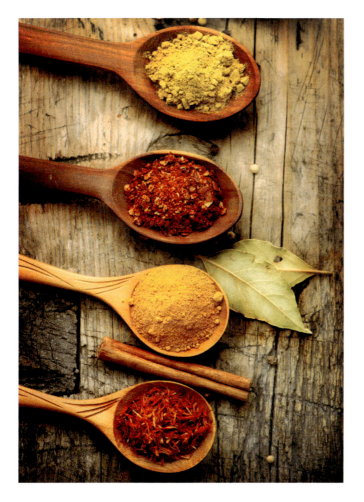

Spoons containing traditional Indian spices. Photo source: subbotina/123rf.com.
(3.15)

The Consultation

During the consultation with your South Asian client, you need to examine their medical history, cultural practices, dietary intake, and home skincare regimen. Also conduct a visual and tactile exam of the skin.

Your intake form should include a Fitzpatrick skin scale identification, and a question asking your client what ethnicity they identify with. Your client may have skin that looks like a Fitzpatrick skin type 3 (olive skin, dark eyes and hair), but their DNA contains the characteristics of South Asian skin, which would be a Fitzpatrick skin type 4, 5 or 6. Treating a client using an incorrect identification of their Fitzpatrick skin type could result in a negative reaction.

Develop a relationship of trust with your client by delving into details during the consultation. Ask your client about their home skincare routine. Are they using a lightening agent? What ingredients are in the product? Do they practice Ayurvedic balancing regimens? Hot yoga can be a trigger for hyperpigmentation, including melasma. If they are Indian American, have they adopted an Americanized diet of processed food? Are they eating foods rich with antioxidants and anti-inflammatory properties? Ask for clarification on anything they have indicated on their health history. Double-check their allergies. What are their goals? Make sure they understand that professional treatments are a process and not an instant fix.

During the physical exam of your client's skin do you notice periocular hyperpigmentation? Do they have evidence of melasma? Look for the signs of PIH. Is their skin sensitive, normal, oily, or combination? Is their skin sensitized from over-exfoliation or the use of harsh products?

Get photos of your client's skin as a baseline for comparison. Get photos in a front view, and side views (fig 3.16).

The Treatment Plan

Your consultation will guide you to the best treatment plan for your client. Offer a treatment plan that is comprehensive and includes professional sessions, as well as the home skincare regimen that they will need to get their skin to a healthy condition. Because of the risks of PIH with an aggressive treatment, you will need to condition your client's skin and build up a tolerance to stronger ingredients and progressively stronger treatments. Recognizing and treating PIH as soon as it is identified will help lessen the severity and length of time the client is dealing with the PIH.

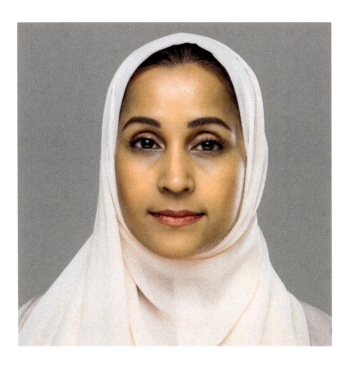

Before photos are a critical component of any treatment plan. Photo source: oneinchpunch/stock.adobe.com.

(3.16)

Microdermabrasion/Infused Microdermabrasion

You need to take a progressive rather than aggressive approach toward your client when performing mechanical exfoliating treatments. Limiting the number of passes in diamond microdermabrasion, or using a mild solution for the infused microdermabrasion until you are familiar with your client's skin reactions, will gradually build your client's skin tolerance, so they can progress to a more aggressive treatment regimen. Finish your treatment with a hydrating mask, and make sure your client has hydrating aftercare products for home.

Chemical Peels

Chemical peels need a very gentle approach with South Asian clients. A possible reaction to a chemical peel is transient hyperpigmentation. Start with an enzyme peel and progress the strength of your peel series. Transition your client to stronger peel applications. When the product is applied, your client should never feel that the discomfort level is above a 5 on a scale of 1 to 10. Because Indian skin is categorized as a Fitzpatrick 5 or 6, the chance for hyperpigmentation is even greater, so a five is the best option. The peel may not ever give your client visible sheets of skin peeling from the skin, but will cause a micro-shedding exfoliation. When your client can tolerate an enzyme peel you can progress to a gentle alpha hydroxy acid peel. Malic acid, mandelic acid, and mid-pH, low-percentage glycolic acid peels are excellent options. Twenty percent glycolic acid was proven effective in a study done by the Department of Aesthetic Medicine in the United Kingdom. A 15% lactic acid mixed with a 3.75% TCA also had positive results lasting four to six months. Salicylic peels respond well with acneic South Asian clients. In a series of peels, increase the strength over a period of months. Do not treat your client immediately with a 20% glycolic acid peel, for example.

Facial Devices

Your South Asian client should have a good response to treatments using microcurrent, ultrasonic and negative ion transmissions. A study in the United Kingdom also demonstrated improvements in under eye circles with a series of microneedling sessions.

Dermaplaning is a nice option for South Asian clients who are not candidates for laser hair removal because of concerns about paradoxical hair growth or no access to the 1064 Nd: YAG for the safest treatment.

With any device, a series of treatments will condition your client's skin and cause gradual improvements. Remind your client that a series of treatments is what will get them results. Be sure to take photos at each session to document the progress.

Lasers and IPL

If your client is requesting hair removal services, make sure they have the opportunity to learn about paradoxical hair growth to make an informed decision. It is a rare side effect, but they need to know the possibilities before committing to a series of treatments.

Consider conditioning your client's skin with melanocyte inhibiting skincare products for four to six weeks prior to beginning a series of skin rejuvenating laser treatments in order to reduce the risk of PIH after a laser session.

Use intense pulsed light (IPL) cautiously and test pulse your client prior to engaging in a full treatment. Observe for a skin reaction that reaches clinical endpoint rather than exceeds clinical endpoint with excessive erythema and edema.

The IPL will continue to work in the skin after the client leaves your treatment room and overexposure could be harmful and initiate a cascade of hyperpigmentation that will be challenging to repair.

Radio frequency collagen induction therapy is gaining in popularity and could be an effective option for your client's skincare needs, but requires caution. Including test pulses to validate your decision to treat will make you confident in your approach toward treatment.

If you are using high powered devices, you need to verify that the device is FDA approved for treating your client's Fitzpatrick skin type.

Combination Treatments

Conditioning your client's skin with melanocyte inhibiting skincare products prior to professional skincare treatments will help reduce the risk of PIH. When working on pigmentation, whether PIH, POH, or melasma, topical applications of skincare products with lightening agents is highly recommended (fig 3.17). Lightening agents can cause skin irritation so it will be a delicate balance for you as a professional to manage the irritating ingredients, which can cause inflammation, with calming ingredients.

Recommending combination treatments is a smart option for your clients. You can titrate the aggressiveness based on your client's responses to previous treatments. Alternating laser treatments, chemical peels, radio frequency, microneedling, as well as mechanical exfoliating sessions will build your client's ability to tolerate more aggressive treatments and reach your client's skincare goals.

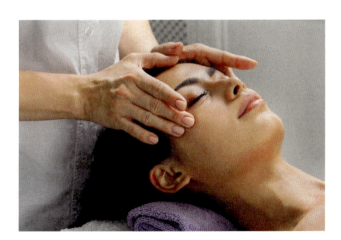

Topical lightening agents will help with hyperpigmentation and condition the skin.
Photo source: milkos/123rf.com.
(3.17)

Home Skincare Recommendations

When you commit to a progressive treatment plan that starts with gentle ingredients, your South Asian client will develop confidence in your skills. Ensure your client that you'll advance their treatment as their skin strengthens.

For pigmentation issues, home care should include a gentle cleanser and pH-balancing toner. An aggressive cleanser could stimulate inflammation in the skin and ultimately fight against the reduction in pigmentation. Start your client on a plant or fungus based melanocyte inhibitor. This will condition their skin to accept a low-dose hydroquinone product for a short therapeutic session. Hydroquinone is a controversial skincare ingredient, but it has a place in treating challenging pigmentation for short-term use. Transition them from 2% hydroquinone to 4% hydroquinone and then back to a plant or fungi based melanocyte inhibitor over a course of six to eight months. Your client should see pigmentation begin to blend, but during times of hot weather, they may have to increase their topical application, or titrate in some topical hydroquinone for a short time again.

Your client may need lighter or heavier hydration depending on if they have oily or dry skin. They may need short term hydration with calming agents if they are sensitized from an aggressive session.

Acne treatments can be successful with the same progressive approach. Common ingredients that are effective against acne, such as benzoyl peroxide, salicylic acid, and retinoic acids, can be effective at thinning the stratum corneum and keeping the follicle open, but you will have to condition your client's skin gradually. Because of its lipophilic properties, some studies have shown South Asian skin responds positively to salicylic acid for acne.

Conclusion

South Asian skin has some unique differences. Being cognizant of the risk of pigmentation issues such as hyperpigmentation, as well as other negative effects, will help you treat South Asian clients properly. A treatment program that starts gently and progressively gets stronger will lower the risk of adverse reactions. Knowing how to treat your South Asian client by understanding their unique needs will empower you as a confident beauty professional who your clients will recognize and trust.

NOTES

1. "Map of Human Migration," *Genographic Project*, accessed March 26, 2019, https://genographic.nationalgeographic.com/human-journey/.

2. Megan Brickley and Rachel Ives, "Chapter 5 - Vitamin D Deficiency," in *The Bioarchaeology of Metabolic Bone Disease*, (Amsterdam: Elsevier Academic Press, 2009), 75-150.

Fig 3.4. "Global Human Journey," *National Geographic*, accessed April 15, 2019, https://www.nationalgeographic.org/media/global-human-journey/educator/.

Fig 3.5. Mohammed Radmanesh, "Paradoxical hypertrichosis and terminal hair change after intense pulsed light hair removal therapy," *Journal of Dermatological Treatment* 20, no. 1 (Jul 2009): 52-54, fig. 1, fig. 2, https://doi.org/10.1080/09546630802178224.

Fig 3.6. Mohammed Alghoul et al., "Eyelid Reconstruction," *Plastic and Reconstructive Surgery* 132, no. 2 (Aug 2013): 288e-302e, https://doi.org/10.1097/PRS.0b013e3182958e6b.

Fig 3.7. Pratik B. Sheth, Hiral A. Shah, and Jayendra N. Dave, "Periorbital hyperpigmentation: A study of its prevalence, common causative factors and its association with personal habits and other disorders," *Indian Journal of Dermatology* 59, no. 2 (2014): 151-157, fig. 5, https://doi.org/10.4103/0019-5154.127675.

Fig 3.8. Sheth, Shah, and Dave, "Periorbital hyperpigmentation," 151-157, fig. 1.

Fig 3.9. Sheth, Shah, and Dave, "Periorbital hyperpigmentation," 151-157, fig. 6.

Fig 3.10. Sheth, Shah, and Dave, "Periorbital hyperpigmentation," 151-157, fig. 7.

Fig 3.11. Adam Jones, *Fair and Lovely - Billboard for Skin-Whitening Cream - Chittagong - Bangladesh*, March 12, 2014, photograph, Flickr, https://www.flickr.com/photos/adam_jones/13103725423/in/photolist-qybU9b-ofkjaY-o8L36G-nBx2fu-8D3p96-k9EAGd-nreCGh-kXW23p-C4tT1Z-AVMdgx-wgD7LN-uAaMtd-k9RxE-quFi6G-8Ffezy-8jq1DS-6Q9BR9-6EisrZ.

https://creativecommons.org/licenses/by-sa/2.0/legalcode

Fig 3.12. Hilary Whiteman, "Vaseline skin-lightening app stirs debate," CNN, July 16, 2010, http://www.cnn.com/2010/WORLD/asiapcf/07/16/facebook.skin.lightening.app/index.html.

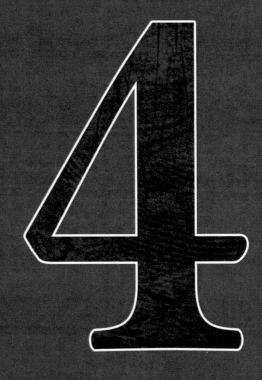

4

INDIGENOUS SKIN

INDIGENOUS SKIN

Kiana is a member of the Tulalip Tribe (fig 4.1). Her people come from what were the Duwamish, Snohomish, Snoqualmie, Ska git, Sauk-Suiattle and Samish tribes. The federal government placed these tribes into one group on a reservation in 1855. This tribe ate a diet rich with seafood, including salmon, shellfish, and clams. Deer, elk, and fowl also contributed to protein in the diet, while berries and roots offered additional nutrients, including healthy antioxidants.[1] A healthy diet contributed to skin health.

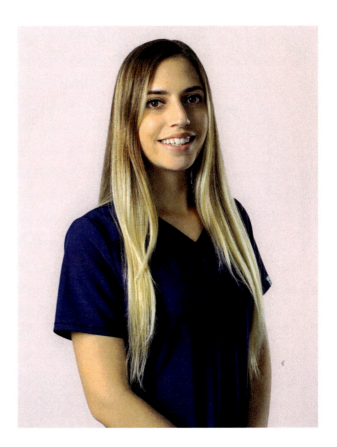

Kiana, a licensed esthetician, entrepreneur and member of the Tulalip Tribe. Photo source: Megan Rayo, Electric Beauty Productions.
(4.1)

In 1860 the United States began a program called 'Kill the Indian, Save the Man' to eradicate Indigenous peoples by requiring children to attend boarding schools and assimilate into American culture. The Tulalip Tribe children were the first residents of St. Anne's Mission, the first Indian school in 1869 (fig 4.2-3). Students had their hair cut, and they were forbidden from speaking their native language. The last boarding schools closed in 1973 when Indigenous people joined the Civil Rights movement demanding autonomy.

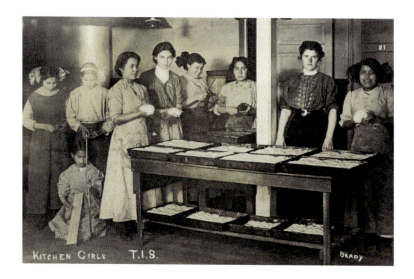

Top Image
Girls working in the kitchen at the Tulalip Indian School, ca. 1912. Every student was required to spend at least half of their day working to assist in the operation of the school. Boys worked as carpenters, engineers, and farmers; girls were assigned to sewing, laundry, and kitchen work. Photo source: MOHAI, Ferdinand Brady Photographic Postcards, 1988.11.16.
(4.2)

Bottom Image
Parents were allowed to visit the school on weekends. This family portrait is of Lucy and Bill Dunbar with their children Josephine and Billy, Jr., who both attended the Tulalip Indian School, ca. 1912. MOHAI, Ferdinand Brady Photographic Postcards, 1988.11.23.
(4.3)

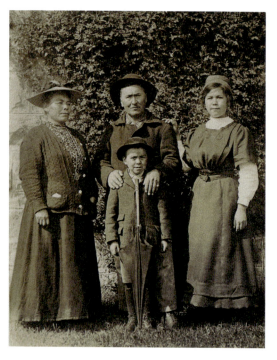

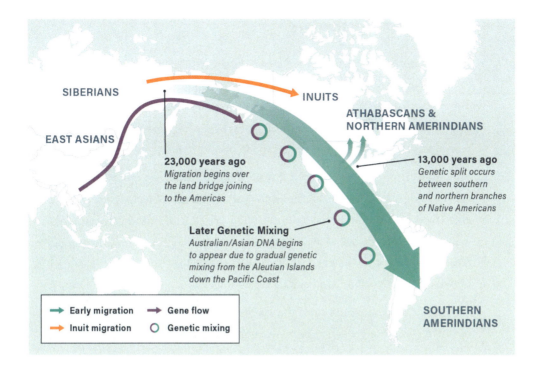

Population of the Americas began 23,000 years ago with Eurasian migration over the Bering Straight land bridge. Scientists attribute the rich genetic diversity found in some populations to a second migration that may have occurred later or via a different route. Map information source: Hoban, "Researches suggest," *The Boston Globe*; map created by: Sarah Jensen.
(4.4)

What Are the Characteristics

Indigenous skin has some similarities with Asian skin due to the prehistoric migration of humans from Africa. American Indigenous people traveled from Asia, across the Bering Strait, 15,000 years ago (fig 4.4).[2]

Additional physiology includes:

- Epicanthic folds
- Incisor teeth with a ledge on the backside[3]
- A gap between the front teeth
- Lingual nodes, or two bony pieces that protrude from the jawbone under the tongue
- A pigmentation in the back of the eye on the retina[4]
- Fewer hair follicles on the body[5]
- Larger number of hair follicles on the scalp[6]
- Fewer eccrine glands[7]

Diseases and Disorders

Indigenous Americans have the highest incidence of diabetes of any ethnic group in the United States. Researchers believe this is due to rapid diet changes with the introduction of European food. Indigenous people had a diet filled with low-glycemic, calorie-dense foods for thousands of years. With the European introduction of refined sugar and other high glycemic foods, obesity and diabetes resulted.[8]

Indigenous Americans also suffer from a higher incidence of thyroid disorders. Anthropologists discovered an Indigenous artifact from 2000 years ago in the Ohio area (fig 4.5). This figure has a goiter. Indigenous tribes used tobacco. Tobacco is known to rob the soil of iodine, a necessary mineral for thyroid function. It is reasoned by the researchers that a glacier's path 300,000 years previous and the growth of tobacco crops depleted the soil of iodine.

Indigenous Americans lack the enzyme needed to convert alcohol in the bloodstream so there is a higher prevalence of alcoholism.[9]

Actinic prurigo an abnormal reaction to sunlight that causes papular or nodular skin eruptions, is thought to be an auto-immune disorder that manifests itself pre-puberty in Indigenous girls, although not exclusively (fig 4.6). It often appears early in the spring in sun-exposed areas of skin. Symptoms include intensely itchy papulonodular lesions with erythema, predominantly on the bridge of the nose, cheeks, and lower lip, although lesions can appear anywhere. Due to the itching, skin excoriations, scarring, and post-inflammatory hyperpigmentation can result.

Acne is another skin condition that modern Indigenous people are experiencing, despite having very little to no acne incidence prior to European diet influences.[10, 11]

Indigenous people also suffer from a high rate of rosacea that can be undiagnosed because symptoms do not look like Nordic rosacea.[12] Flushing and telangiectasias are hard to detect due to the melanin in the skin, and papules can be confused with acne or dermatitis lesions.

Kiana is a passionate skincare professional who plans on opening her own med spa one day in a town along the Columbia River, in what was once a large trading center for Indigenous people. She has been in the service industry since her teens, working as a waitress and then began her own cleaning business. Her passion for esthetics was ignited after she worked for a time as a receptionist at a lash and waxing salon.

Her skin has lightened since her childhood as she has adopted healthier skin practices so she is often mistaken for a Fitzpatrick 2. Her ethnic heritage includes

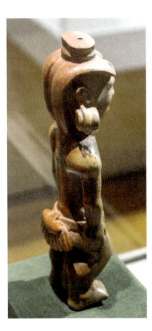
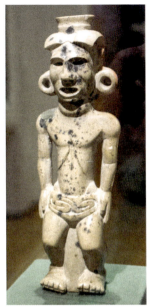

Top Image
Human effigy pipe used for smoking tobacco. Made by the Adena people out of pipestone some time between 100 BC and 100 AD, found at the Adena Mound near Chillicothe, Ohio in 1901. The swollen neck on the figure is suggestive of a goiter. This indicates possible nutrient deficiencies in the person whom after the pipe was fashioned. Photo source: Evanson, *human effigy pipe*.
(4.5)

Bottom Image
An eruption of actinic prurigo on the face characterized by a rash of small, itchy papules. Actinic prurigo primarily affects sun-exposed areas such as the face, neck, and dorsal surfaces of upper extremities. Photo source: Ngan, "Actinic prurigo," DermaNet NZ.
(4.6)

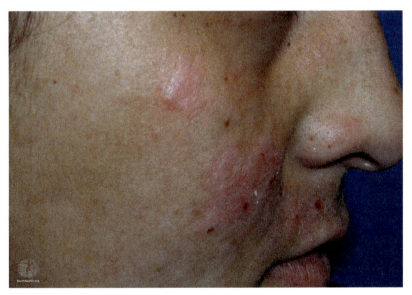

Tulalip tribe as well as Polynesian, Nordic, Black and Latinx so she is extremely aware of the need for accurate Fitzpatrick scale ranking during a consultation.

Kiana is also committed to healthy living after witnessing cancer, alcoholism and rosacea in her family. She understands what these diseases can do to the body and the evidence of their existence through the skin. Her personal experience and her continued education toward an advanced esthetics licensure is preparing her to be a thorough, skilled and compassionate practitioner.

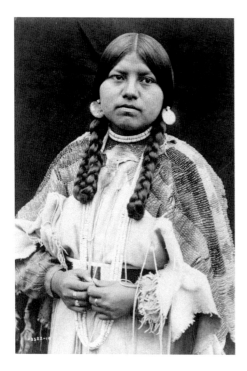
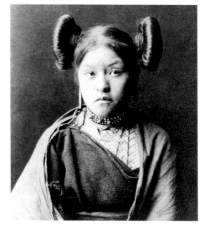

Like languages and belief systems, hair styling practices varied throughout communities across the country. On the left is a Cayuse woman in a ceremonial dress with two long braids. On the right is the "squash blossom whorl," a traditional Hopi hairstyle worn by unmarried girls. Photo source: Library of Congress, Prints & Photographs Division, Edward S. Curtis Collection.
(4.7)

Cultural Practices

Many Indigenous tribes were matriarchal, a stark difference from European patriarchy. Indigenous cultural practices were transferred through art and the oral tradition for thousands of years. Many beauty traditions were lost as Indigenous people were removed from their lands and placed on reservations as well as being forced to assimilate to European culture.

Indigenous people considered hair to be sacred (fig 4.7). It symbolized a connection to all thoughts, experiences, and history. Braiding of hair symbolized the strength of family, tribe, and the connection to all of creation. A single strand of hair is weak, but braided hair becomes strong. Intimate relationships are formed through nurturing activities such as brushing and braiding of hair. Hair was cut to symbolize a significant loss, such as a death, life change, or traumatic event. It was an identifier to the rest of the tribe that the person was in mourning. The cut hair was burned ceremonially rather than just discarded in the trash.

European efforts to assimilate Indigenous peoples included cutting their hair. This act of dominance stripped Indigenous people of their heritage and identity.

It is considered disrespectful today to touch a person's hair, including the hair of children and the elderly. It is considered to be crossing a personal boundary.[13]

The Indigenous peoples of the Great Plains practice skin offerings as a part of the Sun Dance ceremony. Practitioners pierce their chest, back, or arms with wooden sticks as part of a prayer for the welfare of a person's family or the community. Dermatologists unaware of the tradition have diagnosed the skin markings as acne scarring due to severe cystic acne and mistakenly treated them with Accutane®.[14]

Indigenous people used herbs and plants for skin and hair care that are now used in many commercial preparations today (fig 4.8).

Aloe is an almost miracle plant with antimicrobial, antibacterial, antifungal, and anti-inflammatory properties. It provides soothing relief to irritants and contains the antioxidant vitamins A, B, C, D and E, along with minerals zinc, magnesium, and potassium.

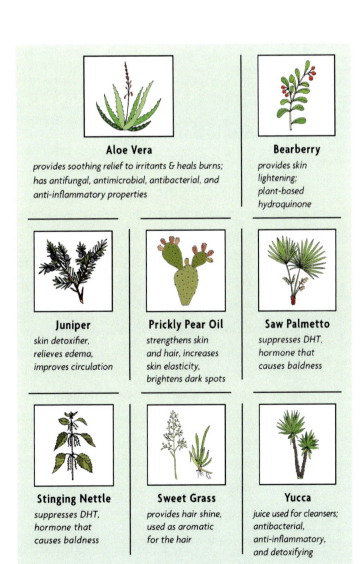

Plants and herbs historically used by Indigenous people for hair and skin care. Graphic source: Foxyliam/Shutterstock.com, edited by Sarah Jensen.

(4.8)

Prickly pear oil was used to help strengthen the skin and hair. The oil contains twice as many proteins and fatty acids as argan oil. It is rich in vitamin E, an antioxidant that helps repair damaged and mature skin. The linoleic and oleic fatty acids in prickly pear oil provide hydration and increase skin elasticity. It also contains vitamin K and is used to brighten dark spots and lighten undereye circles.

Juniper is an important ingredient in balancing oily skin, improving circulation, and relieving edema. It is also a skin detoxifier.

Yucca is antibacterial, anti-inflammatory, and detoxifying. The juice is lathering, so it is used for cleansers. It also contains vitamin C which nourishes the skin.[15]

Saw palmetto and stinging nettle are plants that were dried and ground into a powder. They suppress the hormone DHT (dihydrotestosterone), the cause of baldness.[16]

Bearberry, a plant-based hydroquinone, was used as a skin lightener.

Sweetgrass was used as an aromatic for the hair as well as for its ability to give the hair shine.[17]

The Consultation

The consultation should be where you build trust with your client and become familiar with their skin and aspects of their life that influence their skin (fig 4.9). Review your client's medical history and intake form. Giving the appointment your full attention will result in a better outcome for your client.

A solid skin analysis will help you determine your client's skin type: oily, dry, sensitive, or normal. Does your client have dry, flaky, dull-looking skin or do they battle shininess and congestion?

Cardiac function, digestion, muscle movements, bone development, brain function, and metabolism are dependent on the hormones produced by the thyroid gland. This butterfly shaped gland is at the base of the throat. The thyroid uses iodine from blood to produce thyroid hormones[18]. Does your client suffer from a thyroid disorder? Dry flaking skin is a sign of hypothyroidism, or an underactive thyroid.

Is your client eating a diet of fresh vegetables and fruit and adequate protein, or does their diet contain a high level of processed food? Are they dehydrated?

Are the papulonodular lesions acne or actinic prurigo?

Ask about your client's home care regimen.

Does your client have specific goals? Do they have an event coming up or a special occasion that they are preparing for?

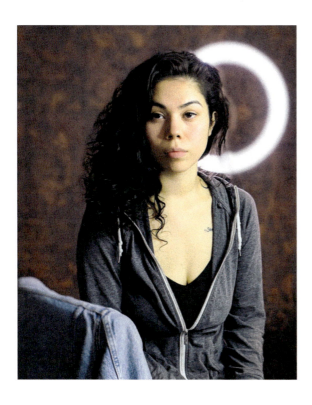

Building trust with your client by spending time in a thorough consultation will increase client loyalty and prevent a negative outcome. Photo source: Obi Onyeador on Unsplash.
(4.9)

Verify your client's allergies. If you will be performing chemical peels, this knowledge will determine the type of peel you select for your client.

Use the Fitzpatrick scale to get a general idea of your client's skin type and how it responds to UV exposure.

It is important to take photos before treatment so you have a baseline for comparison. Take photos from multiple viewpoints.

The Treatment Plan

Take some time to review all the details you have acquired in the consultation before you develop the treatment plan. Any treatment plan will have to consider the repercussions from post-inflammatory hyperpigmentation (PIH).

Skin improvements will be progressive rather than instantaneous, and a slow and steady approach is better than an aggressive approach. Most clients will appreciate your cautiousness and the reassurance that you have their best interests in mind.

Instruct your client on a series of professional treatments as well as a home skincare regimen.

Microdermabrasion/Infused Microdermabrasion

Due to the risk of PIH, begin with a mild microdermabrasion or wet microdermabrasion for the first session. Because removing the stratum corneum allows skincare products to penetrate easily and results in faster efficacy, it's a great approach to introducing home skincare. It is also a great first introduction to other professional treatments. Do not perform microdermabrasion on sensitive skin.

CHEMICAL PEELS	WHAT PEEL DOES	BEST FOR
Glycolic (AHA)	Most common peel. It reduces appearance of fine lines, increases cell turn over rate, removes dead skin cells, and brightens skin.	All skin types; especially those with wrinkles and fine lines
Lactic (AHA)	A less irritating peel. It evens skin tone, lightens pigmentation, reduces appearance of wrinkles and age spots, and can be moisturizing.	All skin types; especially for hyper-pigmented skin, dry/sensitive, and mature skin
Salicylic (BHA)	Penetrates deeper in the skin. It helps control acne, eliminates blackheads and whiteheads, clarifies skin, and reduces pore blockage.	Acne prone and oily skin
Trichloroacetic (TCA)	A medium strength peel. It reduces the appearance of wrinkles, fine lines, acne scars. Good for skin tightening, large pores, and sun damaged skin.	All skin issues, but better for lighter complexions
Fruit Enzyme	Common fruit enzymes are papaya, pineapple, and pumpkin. They promote cell renewal and are anti-bacterial.	Rosacea, dehydrated skin, and sensitive skin

A guide to common chemical peels, their benefits, and recommended skin types. For Indigenous clients always start with an enzyme peel and slowly progress to more aggressive treatments. Chart information source: Petrillo, "A Simple Guide," Perfect Image; created by: Sarah Jensen. (4.10)

Chemical Peels

The first peel should be an enzyme (fig 4.10). If your client can tolerate an enzyme peel, the next peel in the series should be a low-percentage acid with a high pH. Microscopic sloughing of skin is the goal, not visible peeling. Visible skin shedding may indicate the treatment was too aggressive and could result in PIH. You can target pigmentation issues, fine lines, texture, and pore size by using a large molecule AHA alternately with a BHA.

Build your client's skin strength by increasing the percentage of acid or decreasing the pH slightly. With this approach you are exercising your client's skin and slowly increasing your ability to use more aggressive treatments.

Facial Devices

Ultrasonic spatula, high-frequency devices, and galvanic devices are useful tools that may bring improvements to your client's skin when implemented during a facial.

For more invasive treatments, do a skin test first to determine appropriateness. Take hyperpigmentation in consideration when using treatments like microneedling. Begin slowly with a shorter needle depth and fewer passes until you are familiar with your client's skin response.

Lasers and Intense Pulsed Light (IPL)

After your Indigenous client's skin has been conditioned with a series of chemical peels and the home use of a melanin suppressant, fractional laser treatments are an option.

1064 Nd: YAG is considered the gold standard for treating skin of color.

IPL is not a treatment modality for Indigenous skin because of the concentration of melanocytes in the dermis and epidermis.

Although some companies will claim their device is capable of safely treating Fitzpatrick skin types 5 and 6, you must remember that the intense pulsed light energy will be activated in the skin for hours after the treatment, and negative reactions may not be fully visible until the next day.

Radio frequency collagen induction therapy is gaining in popularity and could be an effective option for your client's skincare needs, but caution is needed. Including test pulses will make you confident in your approach toward treatment.

If you are using high-powered devices, you need to verify that the device is FDA approved for treating your client's Fitzpatrick skin type and never exceed the manufacturer's recommended guidelines for settings.

Combination Treatments

Your client can benefit from treatments that approach the skin differently. Alternating modalities can condition your client's skin and build its ability to use stronger acids or device settings; however, the skin must be pretreated with melanocyte inhibitors first to reduce the risk of PIH. Balance your proscribing of skin lighteners containing irritating ingredients with moisturizers that have calming and soothing properties.

LED light therapy is a great combination therapy. Green light can help with pigmentation; red light is anti-aging; and blue light is effective for acne.

Home Skincare Recommendations

Your client may not be familiar with professional skincare when they come to you, so spend time explaining the importance of home care (fig 4.11). Eighty percent of their results will come from the home care that is partnered with the professional treatments. Add products to their home care regimen one at a time, so if they have irritation or inflammation, you can easily recognize which product is causing the problem. You can steadily add more potent ingredients as you become familiar with their skin's reactions and tolerance levels. Beware of harsh ingredients that compromise transepidermal water loss (TEWL) since it may result in rebound oiliness.

As you incorporate ingredients, start your client on a gentle cleanser and pH-balancing toner.

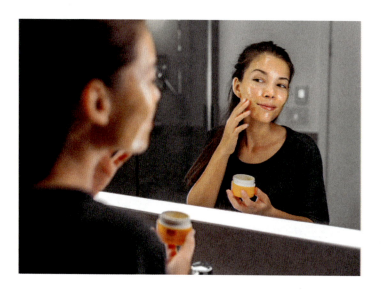

Reinforcing the value of a home skincare regimen during your consultation will help your client see better results from your professional treatments. Photo source: Maridav/Shutterstock.com.
(4.11)

When working with an acneic client, avoid products that are harsh and drying as they can result in rebound oiliness and increased acne breakouts. Low-percentage salicylic acid usually works well due to its antimicrobial properties. Retinol is often recommended as an acne treatment. Your client can get discouraged with use because of its tendency to cause dryness and sensitivity, but it can be started in low dosages and titrated up in concentration and amount as the skin builds tolerance.

Make your moisturizer recommendation based on your skin assessment. Your client may need lighter hydration if their skin is oily and a heavier emollient for dryness.

Introduce serums such as epidermal growth factors and antioxidants slowly to nourish the skin and build collagen, incrementally increasing use from twice weekly for two weeks to three times a week for two weeks to every other day and then finally to daily use.

You may have to introduce sunscreen to your client. They may have the cultural belief that they do not need SPF because they do not get skin cancer.[19] Indigenous Americans die of melanoma at higher percentages than the national average[20] and 50% of Indigenous people with skin cancer will die of the disease compared to other ethnicities.[21]

Conclusion

Gain your client's trust with strong consultation skills, a respect for their culture, and by explaining that treating skin of color is a journey that involves gradual improvements from treatment.

You can treat your Indigenous American client with confidence when you take a progressive rather than aggressive approach.

Elevate your profession by being knowledgeable about all skin types. Indigenous skin has specific needs, and you need to be skilled in treating all ethnicities as our country becomes more multiethnic.

NOTES

1. Margaret Riddle, "Tulalip Tribes," History Link, November 27, 2008, https://historylink.org/File/8852.

2. "Other Migration Theories – Bering Land Bridge National Preserve," Bearing Land Bridge National Preserve Alaska, National Park Service, last modified February 22, 2017, https://www.nps.gov/bela/learn/historyculture/other-migration-theories.htm.

3. "Shovel-shaped incisors," Wikimedia Foundation, last modified July 29, 2020, 00:11, https://en.wikipedia.org/wiki/Shovel-shaped_incisors.

4. Pathways thru life, "My Cherokee Heritage and General Cherokee History," We Have Kids, updated February 6, 2019, https://wehavekids.com/family-relationships/Cherokee-Heritage.

5. Phillip Milano, "Dare To Ask: Native Americans and body hair," *The Florida Times-Union*, July 29, 2009, https://www.jacksonville.com/lifestyles/columnists/phillip_milano/2009-07-29/story/dare_to_ask_do_native_americans_have_facial_an.

6. Marie Miguel, "5 Reasons Natives Have Lustrous Locks: Ancient, Indigenous Hair Remedies," Indian Country Today, May 29, 2017, https://indiancountrytoday.com/archive/5-reasons-natives-have-lustrous-locks-ancient-indigenous-hair-remedies-pDXtTkdyNUSbdVyviFZLfQ.

7. Catherine Lu and Elaine Fuchs, "Sweat Gland Progenitors in Development, Homeostasis, and Wound Repair," *Cold Spring Harbor Perspectives in Medicine* 4, no. 2 (Feb 2014): a015222, https://doi.org/10.1101/cshperspect.a015222.

8. Stephanie Pappas, "Feces Fossil Sheds Light on Native Americans' High Diabetes Risk," Huffington Post, last modified December 6, 2017, https://www.huffpost.com/entry/feces-fossil-native-americans-diabetes-epidemic_n_1701404.

9. Cindy L. Ehlers and Ian R. Gizer, "Evidence for a Genetic Component for Substance Dependence in Native Americans," *American Journal of Psychiatry* 170, no. 2 (February 2013): 154-164, https://doi.org/10.1176/appi.ajp.2012.12010113.

10. Erica C. Davis and Valerie D. Callender, "A Review of Acne in Ethnic Skin: Pathogenesis, Clinical Manifestations, and Management Strategies," *The Journal of Clinical and Aesthetic Dermatology* 3, no. 4 (April 2010): 24-38, https://pubmed.ncbi.nlm.nih.gov/20725545/.

11. Elise May, "Why Indigenous People Don't Have Acne," Skin Nutritious, November 4, 2019, https://skinutritious.com/blogs/articles/why-indigenous-people-dont-have-acne.

12. Damian McNamara, "Skin of Color May Mask Classic Signs of Rosacea," *Family Practice News*, March 15, 2005, https://www.mdedge.com/familymedicine/article/25342/dermatology/skin-color-may-mask-classic-signs-rosacea.

13. Barbie Stensgar, "The Significance of Hair in Native American Culture," *News from the Sisters* (blog), Sister Sky, January 4, 2019, https://sistersky.com/blogs/sister-sky/the-significance-of-hair-in-native-american-culture.

14. Allison Truong, Jillian W. Wong, and Anne Lynn S. Chang, "Native American Skin Offerings Mistaken for Acne Scars in a College Undergraduate," *Arch Dermatol.*, 148, no. 10 (October 2012): 1214-1215, https://doi.org/10.1001/archdermatol.2012.592.

15. Sherrie Strausfogel, "5 Native American Beauty Secrets," Better Nutrition, last modified August 6, 2019, https://www.betternutrition.com/natural-living/native-american-beauty-secrets.

16. Marie Miguel, "5 Reasons Natives Have Lustrous Locks: Ancient, Indigenous Hair Remedies," Indian Country Today, May 29, 2017, https://indiancountrytoday.com/archive/5-reasons-natives-have-lustrous-locks-ancient-indigenous-hair-remedies-pDXtTkdyNUSbdVyviFZLfQ.

17. "Native American Skincare Traditions of Yesterday and Today," *Beauty Blog* (blog), My AlpStory, November 9, 2018, https://alpsglamour.com/native-american-skincare-traditions-of-yesterday-and-today/.

18. "Thyroid gland," You & Your Hormones, accessed August 5, 2020, https://www.yourhormones.info/glands/thyroid-gland/.

19. Melody Maarouf et al., "Skin Cancer Epidemiology and Sun Protection Behaviors Among Native Americans," *J Drugs Dermatol.*, 18, no. 5 (May 2019): 420-423, https://pubmed.ncbi.nlm.nih.gov/31141849/.

20. Tanya H. Lee, "Skin cancer: No one is immune," Indian Country Today, October 21, 2009, https://indiancountrytoday.com/archive/skin-cancer-no-one-is-immune-6QEfPJHGyU2wb2Wz9QCKBQ.

21. Mary E. Logue et al., "Skin Cancer Risk Reduction Behaviors Among American Indian and Non-Hispanic White Persons in Rural New Mexico," *JAMA Dermatol.*, 152, no. 12 (December 2016): 1382-1383, https://doi.org/10.1001/jamadermatol.2016.3280.

Fig 4.2. Ferdinand Brady, *Kitchen Girls, Tulalip Indian School, ca. 1912 - MOHAI 88.11.16*, 1912, Silver gelatin print, Museum of History and Industry, Seattle, https://digitalcollections.lib.washington.edu/digital/collection/loc/id/40.

Fig 4.3. Ferdinand Brady, Family Portrait, *Tulalip Indian School, ca. 1912 - MOHAI 88.11.23*, 1912, Silver gelatin print, Museum of History and Industry, Seattle, https://digitalcollections.lib.washington.edu/digital/collection/loc/id/39.

Fig 4.4. Virgie Hoban, "Researchers suggest another ancestry for Native Americans," *The Boston Globe*, July 21, 2015, https://www.bostonglobe.com/metro/2015/07/21/harvard-study-sheds-new-light-origin-native-american-populations/NTs5hr06ffoq8cWM0T3BGN/story.html.

Fig 4.5. Tim Evanson, *human effigy pipe 01 - Cleveland Museum of Art*, September 23, 2016, photograph, Flickr, https://www.flickr.com/photos/timevanson/30739647306/in/photostream/.

Tim Evanson, *human effigy pipe 02 - Cleveland Museum of Art*, September 23, 2016, photograph, Flickr, https://www.flickr.com/photos/timevanson/30140705483/in/photostream/.
https://creativecommons.org/licenses/by-sa/2.0/

Fig 4.6. Vanessa Ngan, "Actinic prurigo," DermNet NZ, 2006, https://dermnetnz.org/topics/actinic-prurigo/.
https://creativecommons.org/licenses/by-nc-nd/3.0/nz/

Fig 4.7. Edward S. Curtis, *Cayuse woman, half-length portrait, standing, facing front, braids, shell disk earrings, shell bead choker and shell beads around neck, beaded buckskin dress with beaded belt*, ca. 1910, Photographic print, Library of Congress, https://www.loc.gov/item/94504764/.

Edward S. Curtis, *Gobuguoy, Walpi girl, half-length portrait, facing front, hair tied in swirls on sides of head, metal bead and bell choker, printed cotten dress, cotton shawl around shoulders*, ca. 1900, Photographic print, Library of Congress, https://www.loc.gov/item/93501149/.

Fig 4.9. Obi Onyeador, *Native American Woman in a hoodie Sitting in front of a ring light and rust colored background*, 2020, Photograph, Unsplash, https://unsplash.com/photos/wudE2k8bd3k.

Fig 4.10. David Petrillo, "A Simple Guide to Acid Peels," Perfect Image, March 1, 2017, https://perfectimage.com/about/blog/simple-guide-acid-peels/.

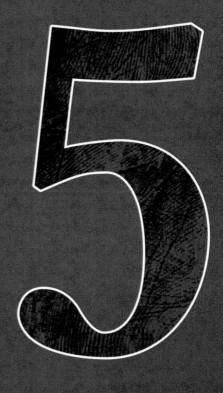

5

LATINX SKIN

LATINX SKIN

Jessie is of Nicaraguan heritage (fig 5.1). Her childhood nickname was "Tostada," meaning "toast." She has darker skin than other family members due to her mixed ancestry. Despite a family culture of "macho" masculine dominance, beauty traditions were handed down from her mother. Misconceptions like not needing sunscreen were perpetuated, along with healthier habits like skin cleaning and nourishing. As Jessie becomes more educated on skin health, she helps our profession find ways to reach out to Latinx consumers.

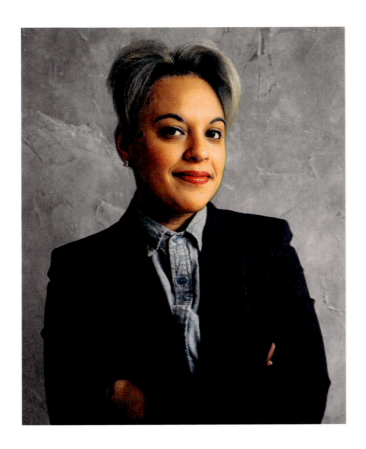

Jessie, proud of her Latinx heritage.
Photo source: Megan Rayo, Electric Beauty Productions.
(5.1)

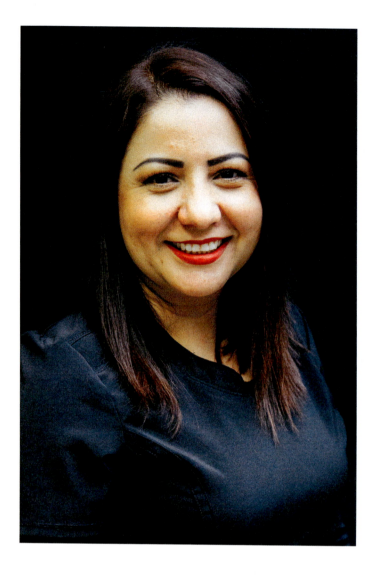

Elva, proud of her Ecuadorean heritage. Photo source: Megan Rayo, Electric Beauty Productions.
(5.2)

Elva grew up in Ecuador (fig 5.2). She is proud of her birthplace and proud of her strong personality that didn't acquiesce to the male-dominant culture. Her mother worked as a seamstress making uniforms and wanted Elva to join her in the business when she grew up. Elva believed she would never marry, relishing the idea of independence. Then she met a man who surprised her by valuing her determination and self reliance, and they got married. They moved to the United States when her husband was offered a teaching position at a college. She had always been attracted to fashion, makeup, hair and skincare since childhood. Her husband encouraged her to pursue her dream by becoming licensed in aesthetics. She hopes to return to Ecuador one day and open her own skincare clinic. Elva is undergoing training on treating Latinx skin in order to provide the best care for her clients.

Latinx identity is often stereotyped as one monochromatic group of people. Latinx is very broad and racially diverse. It is not the same as Hispanic, as Hispanic refers to people of Spanish-speaking origin. Latinx refers to people who originate from the geographical region known as Latin America. Brazil is a part of Latin America so Brazilians are Latinx, but Brazil's official language is Portuguese so they are not Hispanic.[1] A person may be Hispanic but not Latinx or Latinx but not Hispanic.

The US Census added Latino/Latina/Latinx as a racial choice in its 1980 census after a tremendous amount of pressure from Latinx groups. Prior to that, Latinx and Hispanic people were counted as "white" in the US census.

Historically, Latinx civilization extended from South America north through Mexico and into the southwestern United States, where it blended with Indigenous American cultures (fig 5.3). Latinx civilization has had many cultural influences including Spanish colonialism, African slavery, and Native-American culture. It's not one skin type or race. A community may have common language and shared histories but a wide variety of skin colors. Latin America involves many countries and nationalities.

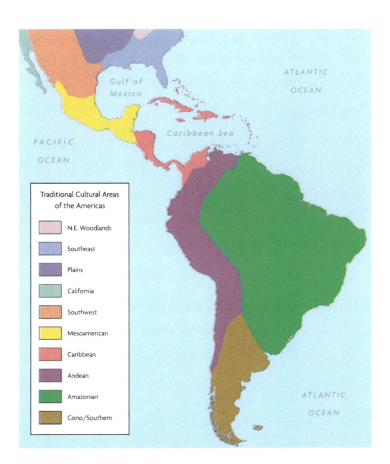

A map showing the traditional areas of Indigenous cultures in Latin America.[2] Map source: Peter Hermes Furian/stock.adobe.com, edited by: Sarah Jensen.

(5.3)

What Are the Characteristics

Latinx skin has its own unique characteristics. These include the following:

- Mast cells are cells formed in our bone marrow that secrete histamines to fight inflammation and provide immune protection. Latinx skin has more granular mast cells so oftentimes it can recover from exposure to irritants more quickly.
- Latinx skin has greater transepidermal water loss (TEWL), like Asian skin.
- Latinx skin has greater melanosome concentration in the basal layer meaning a greater chance of developing post-inflammatory hyperpigmentation (PIH) with injury to the skin.
- Latinx skin can scar easily and may be more likely to form keloids (fig 5.4). Keloids are an overgrowth of scar tissue.[3]

Diseases and Disorders

- Latinxs have a higher incidence of diabetes, which can greatly affect the skin. Diabetes can affect blood flow to the skin due to the body's inability to properly utilize glucose or sugar. Poor blood flow will affect collagen formation, and the skin becomes thinner and drier. Injuries heal more slowly, and the lowered immune response can mean a higher incidence of fungal or bacterial infections.
- Melasma is reported to be as high as 80% in pregnant Mexican women (fig 5.5).[4] Melasma can develop from hormonal influences, but in Latinx skin, melasma can be triggered by injuries to the skin such as acne, rashes, or burns.[5]
- Latinx skin is not more prone to acne, but when a Latinx person develops acne, it may be more cystic. Cystic acne can cause PIH when healing. Although, benzoyl peroxide is a common ingredient in skincare formulated to treat acne, Latinx skin has a sensitivity to benzoyl peroxide, and the effects can be extreme dryness and irritation.[6]
- Skin cancer is on the rise in the Latinx community, and it's likely to be in a later stage when discovered. This is partly due to a cultural falsehood that Latinxs don't get skin cancer. Early symptoms are ignored, and by the time medical attention is sought, the cancer has progressed.

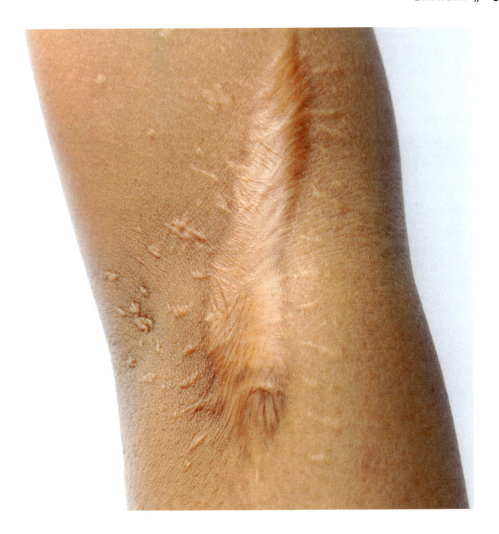

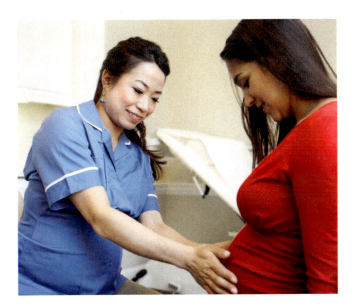

Top Image
Latinx skin is prone to hypertrophic or keloid scarring with injury. Photo source: keawamornmontree/123rf.com.
(5.4)

Bottom Image
Hispanic women risk higher incidence of melasma with pregnancy. Photo source: Mark Bowden/123rf.com.
(5.5)

- Latinx facial muscles display less movement, forming less expressive wrinkles around the eyes, the forehead, and between the brows. This minimizes the wrinkles in aging.[7]

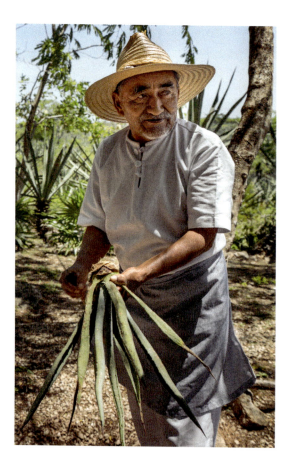

A farmer harvesting an agave plant. Agave has antiseptic properties and has traditionally been used to treat burn, bruises, and minor injuries. Photo source: Leon Rafael/Shutterstock.com.
(5.6)

Cultural and Dietary Practices

Latinx people have a strong culture of self-care due to a tradition of sharing knowledge and the passing down of plant-based medicine (fig 5.6). Occasionally there is a mistrust of professional institutions that may result in medical attention being delayed or avoided.

The Latinx culture is vast, including many countries and unique traditions. Beauty practices vary significantly from culture to culture. In Latinx cultures where female role models are strong, a Latina will have the influences of her mother and other strong women in her life.

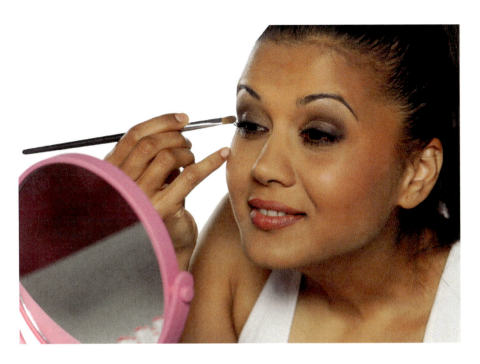

Latinx beauty culture includes self-care time to look your best. Photo source: Vladimir Gjorgiev/123rf.com.

(5.7)

Beauty standards include enhancing feminine features with deep lip color, dark eyeliner, and big hair (fig 5.7). Skincare professionals are esteemed members of society as they provide Latinxs with healthy skin options.

Latinx culture has some biases in its communities in favor of lighter-skinned Latinxs. Studies show that Latinxs with lighter skin have higher-paying jobs, higher education, and are considered more successful. This is a holdover from Spanish occupation and slavery.[8]

The American Latinx is looking for inclusivity and rejects the stereotypical loud, brassy, over-sexualized caricature. Hispanic or Latinx celebrity product endorsements are very influential. Latinxs are educated consumers and make smart choices in skincare and professional skincare services.

Latinx food is often corn-based with corn flour used for tacos, tamales, and tortillas. Tomatoes and other antioxidant-rich vegetables, as well as beans make up a healthy diet. There is a prevailing concept that all Latinx food is spicy. Many foods are flavored with native chiles, but not all food is spicy. Foods are prepared with a variety of subtle flavors. The biggest difference in American meals and Latinx meals is time. Latinxs are more intentional with meal preparation and time spent eating the meal in a social situation. Traditional Latinx culture has not embraced the American fast food indulgence of eating on the run.

As Latinx-American millennials adapt to American mealtime culture, new health issues of obesity and heart disease are growing concerns.

The Consultation

During consultation with your Latinx client, you must consider their medical history, cultural practices, dietary intake, and home skincare regimen, as well as perform a visual and tactile exam of the skin.

Your intake form should include a Fitzpatrick skin scale identification and a question asking your client their ethnic identity. For best treatment, you need to determine the skin color of their family members. Your client may have skin that looks like a Fitzpatrick skin type 3 (olive skin, dark eyes and hair), but their DNA contains the characteristics of Black Latinx skin or Indigenous-American Latinx skin, which would be a Fitzpatrick skin type 5 or 6. Avoid an adverse reaction by taking the time to accurately determine your client's Fitzpatrick skin type.

Dig into the details during your consultation. Does your client have diabetes, and are they taking any diabetic medications to control their blood sugar? Has your client ever had a reaction to a skincare product or ingredient? What allergies do they have? What is their skincare regimen at home? Is their diet one of native Latinx foods, or have they incorporated American foods into their meals? Your client will respect your professional approach when you ask for clarification and reiterate their skincare goals. Because PIH is a concern, make sure they understand that professional treatments will be a process as you work to condition their skin.

During the physical exam, determine if they have evidence of melasma. Look for the signs of PIH. Is their skin sensitive, normal, oily, or combination? Are they struggling with cystic acne? Observe for precancerous lesions.

Get photos of your client's skin as a baseline for comparison. Get photos in a front view, and side views.

The Treatment Plan

Your consultation will guide you to the best treatment plan for your client. Offer a treatment plan that is comprehensive and includes professional sessions, as well as the home skincare that they will need to get their skin to a healthy condition. Because of the risks of PIH with aggressive treatment, you will need to condition your client's skin and build up a tolerance to progressively stronger ingredients and treatments.[9] Recognizing and treating PIH as soon as it is identified, will help lessen the severity and length of recovery. Also understanding that aggressive treatments can affect the acid-mantle balance and increase the risk of fungal and bacterial infections, something your client is already susceptible to, should be taken into consideration.

Microdermabrasion/Infused Microdermabrasion

Latinx skin generally responds well to mechanical exfoliation. Microdermabrasion can help with clogged pores and excess dead skin build-up. Start conservatively in your treatments and build your client's tolerance to more aggressive sessions. Becoming familiar with your client's skin response will help prevent PIH. Latinx skin responds well to masks so nourish your client's skin with a hydrating mask after an exfoliating treatment. Make sure your client has hydrating after care products for home use.

Chemical Peels

Chemical peels are not a go-to solution for Latinx skin. The skin reaction is unpredictable and the chemical process can be too harsh.[10] Aggressive peels can cause transient hyperpigmentation, as well as hypo-pigmentation. A very slow progression of chemical peels with the right acids may benefit your client's skin, but you must proceed cautiously and increase the acid percentage very slowly.

Before starting with a glycolic acid peel, try conditioning your client's skin with lactic, mandelic, malic, or kojic acid peels.

Facial Devices

Latinx skin responds well to microneedling and radio frequency for skin rejuvenation.[11] With any treatment, a series of sessions will condition your client's skin and cause gradual improvements.

Dermaplaning may also be a good option for Latinx clients who are interested in exfoliation.

Take photos at each appointment and review with your client so they can see the incremental changes.

Lasers and IPL

Fractional laser treatments work well with Latinx skin. Begin your client on a home regimen of melanocyte inhibiting skincare for four to six weeks prior to the laser treatments to reduce the chances of rebound PIH. Fractional devices will have a faster recovery with less erythema and edema.

IPL is a risky treatment modality for Latinx skin because of the concentration of melanocytes in the dermis and epidermis. Test pulse your client prior to committing

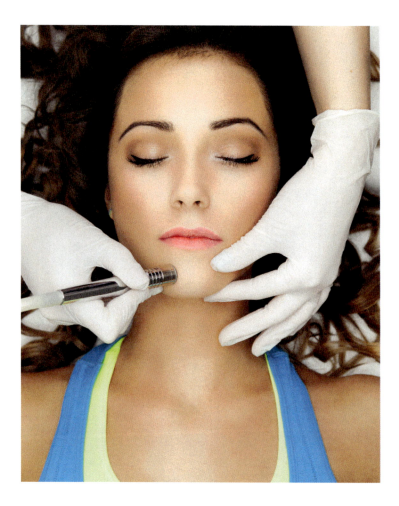

Latinx skin responds well to combination treatments. Photo source: ninamalyna /123rf.com.
(5.8)

to a full treatment. The intense pulsed light energy will be activated in the skin for hours after treatment, and negative reactions may not be fully visible until the next day. IPL should never be used to treat melasma in any Fitzpatrick skin type.

Radio frequency collagen induction therapy is gaining in popularity and could be an effective option for your client's skincare needs. Using caution by including test pulses will make you confident in your approach toward treatment.

If you are using high-powered devices, you need to verify that the device is FDA approved for treating your client's Fitzpatrick skin type, and never exceed the manufacturer's recommended guidelines for settings.

Combination Treatments

Pretreating your client's skin with skincare that inhibits melanin production before beginning a series of treatments, and continuing your client on melanin inhibitors will reduce the risk of hyperpigmentation. You will have to balance your recommendations of skin lighteners that cause irritation with moisturizers that have calming and soothing properties.

Your client will benefit from combination treatments that approach skin problems from different angles (fig 5.8). Alternating treatment modalities with the tools in your aesthetic toolbox, such as fractional laser sessions, mild chemical peels, radio frequency, microneedling session, and mechanical exfoliation will strengthen your client's skin.

Home Skincare Recommendations

Using gentle ingredients when first working with your client will help build trust in your skills. You can gradually add more potent ingredients as you become familiar with their skin's reactions and tolerance levels. Harsh ingredients that compromise barrier function ought to be avoided.

Start your client on a gentle cleanser and pH-balancing toner. Address any pigmentation with a plant or fungus-based melanin inhibitor. You can recommend hydroquinone for short-term use by titrating the strength from 2% to 4% and then back down. Resume a non-hydroquinone product for a daily regimen. In times of hot weather, or if hormones are fluctuating, you may need to resume a short-term use of hydroquinone to bring the melanin production under control. Make your moisturizer recommendation based on your skin assessment. Your client may need lighter hydration if they have oily skin or heavier hydration for dryness.

Latinx skin responds well to epidermal growth factors and antioxidant serums. Use them to nourish the skin and build collagen.

When working with an acneic client, avoid benzoyl peroxide. Salicylic acid and retinols work well. Start slowly and incorporate professional treatments such as LED blue light therapy to control *p. acnes* bacteria.

Conclusion

Latinx is not a race, but an ethnicity that covers a variety of skin colors, nationalities, and geographical influences. Understanding your Latinx client's distinctive skin features is vital, along with Latinx skincare needs including specific diseases and disorders of concern. Ingredient selection is important to ensure an effective treatment plan. Latinxs are one of the fastest growing consumer groups in the United States. You'll develop respect with your Latinx clientele if you treat Latinx skin with the respect it deserves.

NOTES

1. Victoria M. Massie, "Latino and Hispanic Identities Aren't the Same. They're Also Not Racial Groups," *Vox*, September 18, 2016, accessed March 26, 2019, https://www.vox.com/2016/8/28/12658908/latino-hispanic-race-ethnicity-explained.

2. "Native American Indian Culture Areas," Native Languages of the Americas, accessed April 19, 2019, http://www.native-languages.org/culture-areas.htm.

3. Rachel Nall, "Keloid Scar of Skin," *Healthline*, August 9, 2017, accessed March 26, 2019, https://www.healthline.com/health/keloids.

4. "Understanding skin, How does skin differ by ethnic group?," Eucerin, accessed March 26, 2019, https://int.eucerin.com/about-skin/basic-skin-knowledge/skin-ethnics.

5. "Latin/Hispanic Skin," Cosmetic Laser Dermatology Skin Specialists in San Diego, accessed March 26, 2019, https://clderm.com/procedure/latin-hispanic-skin/.

6. "Latin/Hispanic Skin," Cosmetic Laser Dermatology Skin Specialists in San Diego, accessed March 26, 2019, https://clderm.com/procedure/latin-hispanic-skin/.

7. Patricia Reynoso, "An Expert Reveals Why Latina Skin Ages So Well," *Glamour*, May 26, 2017, https://www.glamour.com/story/why-latina-skin-doesnt-age-as-quickly.

8. Giselle Castro, "Why Understanding Colorism Within the Latino Community Is So Important," *HipLatina*, July 31, 2018, https://hiplatina.com/colorism-within-the-latino-community/.

9. Stephanie Nouveau et al., "Skin Hyperpigmentation in Indian Population: Insights and Best Practice," *Indian Journal of Dermatology* 65, no. 5 (Sep-Oct 2016): 487-495, https://www.ncbi.nlm.nih.gov/pmc/articles/PMC5029232/.

10. "Latina Skin Care Guide," Healthy Skin Portal, accessed March 26, 2019, http://www.healthyskinportal.com/articles/latina-skin-care-guide/255/.

11. Michele Sullivan, "Lasers for Latino Skin – A Balance of Gentleness and Strength." *MDedge Dermatology*, March 22, 2017, https://www.mdedge.com/dermatology/article/134023/aesthetic-dermatology/lasers-latino-skin-balance-gentleness-and-strength.

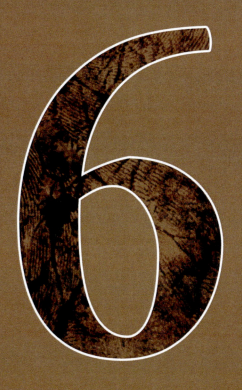

6

NORDIC SKIN

NORDIC SKIN

Nordic skin originated in Scandinavia, Ireland, and Greenland. In other words, Nordic skin is Viking skin. Vikings are explorers and adventurers. They have a fierce spirit, and they also have some distinct anatomical identifying markers.

Mary was born in a tiny town in Minnesota (fig 6.1). The town's population was purely Scandinavian; people immigrated from Sweden, Norway, Denmark and Finland. Her introduction to beauty was watching her mother prepare for an evening out at the local Moose Lodge.

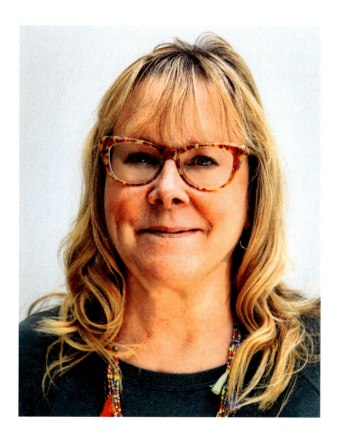

Mary Nielsen, Viking heritage, author. Photo source: Megan Rayo, Electric Beauty Productions.
(6.1)

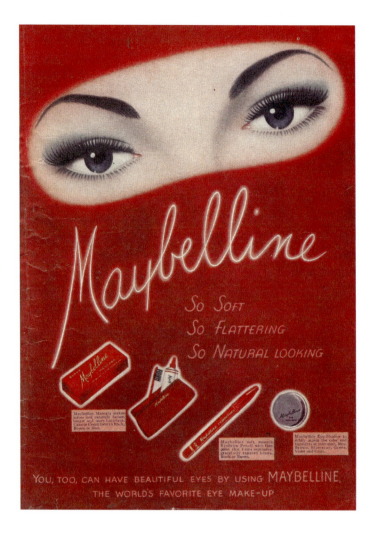

Maybelline magazine ad from 1946.
Photo source: Williams, "Maybelline,"
The Maybelline Story.
(6.2)

As a first-generation American, Mary's mother eschewed the natural beauty look of Nordic culture and sided with the Hollywood celebrity, Elizabeth Taylor. Thick black eyeliner was laid on top of robin-egg-blue eye shadow. Maybelline was the brand of choice (fig 6.2).[1]

Growing up, sunscreen was not even a consideration. But her mother never let her leave the house without a dousing in mosquito repellent.

Sarah's diligence with sunscreen comes from seeing the harsh effects the sun can do to the skin (fig 6.3). Raised on a farm in the Midwest where hard work and simple living were valued, the faces of her family members showed sun damage, deep lines, and early aging due to an absence of SPF sunscreen while engaged in daily outdoor activities. Her Mennonite faith also discouraged any beauty enhancements, so the occasional use of Mary Kay products was the extent of any makeup application. A generational family farm, Sarah could see her grandmother taking the time to curl her own hair, which was unusual for her other female family members. Now that she is in her nineties, Grandma has since adopted the habit of weekly hair appointments at the local beauty salon. Sarah remains true to her Danish heritage with healthy eating habits, frequent outdoor activities, and an uncomplicated beauty regimen of cleansing and SPF application. She allows her natural beauty to shine through with her engaging smile.

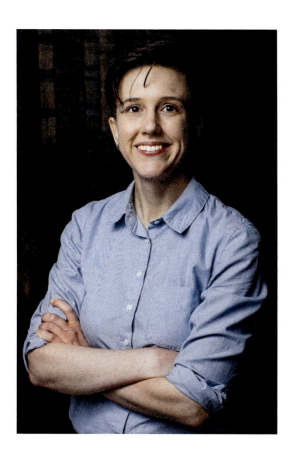

Sarah Jensen, Danish heritage, graphic designer. Photo source: Megan Rayo, Electric Beauty Productions.
(6.3)

What Are the Characteristics

Three primary biological substances determine skin color in all people: melanin in the epidermis, carotene in the dermis, and hemoglobin in the dermal capillaries.

Due to human evolution, people farthest from the equator, developed very pale skin, particularly in the northernmost areas of Europe and Asia (fig 6.4).[2] They did not need nearly as much melanin to protect them from ultraviolet radiation (UV) as equatorial populations. They also needed to absorb UVB more readily in order to produce sufficient vitamin D in regions where daylight could be limited. For instance, in Sweden during January, the sun rises around 8:45 A.M. and sets around 2:55 P.M.

Nordic people have distinct features, but Viking exploration brought diversity to the region.[3] "Black Irish" describes Irish people who are of Irish descent but have black hair and dark eyes.

Nordic features include:

- Fair, pale, or ivory skin corresponding to Fitzpatrick skin types 1 and 2
- Blue eyes
- Blonde or red hair
- Thin skin
- Ages faster

Diseases and Disorders

- A greater chance of developing skin cancer. Globally, Sweden ranks 4th and Norway ranks 5th highest in incidence of skin cancer.[4] Thinner skin and lack of melanin production are contributing factors.
- Scars heal well.
- Bruising is more visible.
- A much higher incidence of sarcoidosis. Sarcoidosis is an autoimmune disorder that causes the formation of granulomas or unusual non-cancerous growths on the skin.[5] They are usually a collection of inflammation that will manifest with more than twenty types of lesions. A referral to a medical professional is your best option when you encounter unfamiliar skin growths.
- Ichthyosis prematurity syndrome is a skin disease that causes thick, dry skin that feels scaly. This disease is caused by a mutation that is almost exclusively found in Norwegians.[6]
- Rosacea was once called the "Curse of the Celts[7]," and its prevalence seems to validate the medical opinion that there is a genetic component to this skin disorder characterized by chronic inflammation that progresses from slight erythema to acneic like pustular breakouts (fig 6.5). If severe, there is skin thickening around the nose.

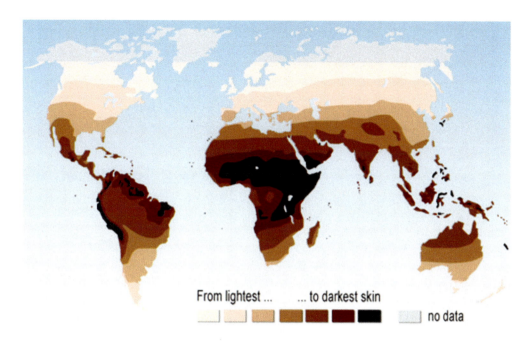

World-wide distribution of human skin color, predicted from multiple environmental factors. Map updated in 2007. Map source: Chaplin, "Geographic Distribution," 292-302, fig 3.
(6.4)

Rosacea is a common skin condition that causes redness and visible blood vessels in the face. It most commonly affects middle-aged women with fair skin and is often mistaken for acne or other skin conditions. Photo source: Milan Lipowski/stock.adobe.com.
(6.5)

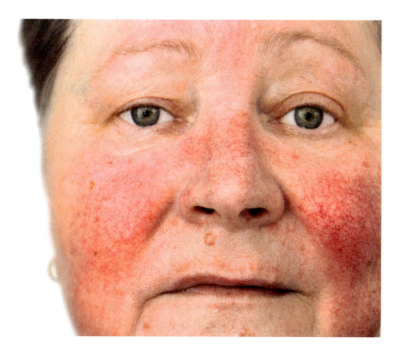

Cultural and Dietary Practices

The Vikings have a reputation for being unkempt heathens, but anthropologists credit Vikings with inventing the first comb (fig 6.6).[8] Archaeological digs have found writings that reference weekly bathing as well as hair and body grooming habits (fig 6.7). The grooming habits are thought to be a way to deal with lice and other vermin that infest the skin and hair.

The Nordic diet is one of the healthiest in the world.[9] A diet full of fish rich in omega-3 fatty acids, root vegetables, and whole grain breads may be one reason why Nordic people are heart healthy and have little acne.

Nordic beauty culture is simplistic with an emphasis on healthy eating and outdoor activities, and there is a similarly minimalistic approach to skincare and makeup. Most Nordic women prefer to wear eyeliner and lipstick only. Antioxidant skin protection is often made from plant based resources, such as cloudberries, which are unique to the geographical region.[10]

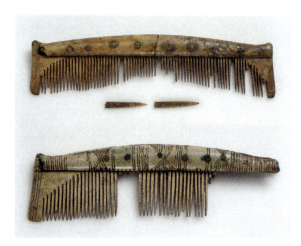

Top Image
Combs made of bone and/or antler from the exhibition "We Call them Vikings" produced by The Swedish History Museum. Photo source: Hildebrandt, *Comb bone*, The Swedish History Museum.
(6.6)

Bottom Image
Bronze tweezers found in a grave from the exhibition "We Call them Vikings" produced by The Swedish History Museum. Photo source: *Tweezers*, The Swedish History Museum.
(6.7)

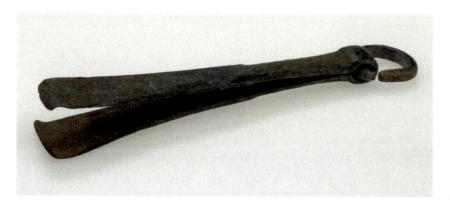

The Consultation

When you sit down with your Nordic client for a consultation, you must consider their medical history, cultural practices, dietary intake, lifestyle, and home skincare regimen. You must also perform a visual and tactile exam of the skin.

If your client has indicated anything on their health history, verbally go over those points. It is important to ask questions regarding any allergies or sensitivities. You need to find out if your client has a family history of rosacea, since their skin may be more fragile and sensitive.

Does your client take any prescription medication related to their skin?

Does your client have issues with dryness due to transepidermal water loss (TEWL)? Thinner dry skin may have impaired barrier function.

Get a clear understanding of your client's lifestyle. What is their skincare budget? Are they committed to a multi-step home care process, or do they need something more straightforward?

In your physical exam of the skin, be sure to evaluate your client's skin thickness and elasticity as well as sun damage and texture. Observe the skin carefully for any abnormal pigmentation or scaly lesions that could signify skin cancer or pre-cancer. Don't be hesitant about referring your client to a medical professional for clearance to continue aesthetic treatments.

By spending time in the consultation and demonstrating you understand the issues that they are trying to correct or improve, you will develop trust with your client and can get a treatment plan.

Make sure that your client understands that a treatment plan will include regularly scheduled visits that compliment the results they will be achieving with home skincare.

Get photos of your client's skin as a baseline for comparison. Get photos in a front view, and side views.

The Treatment Plan

Your client may need treatment options that build collagen and strengthen the skin. With thinner skin, your client may have visible telangiectasias, especially around the nose. Your consultation will guide you to the best treatment plan for your client. Depending on your client's skin sensitivity, you may be able to pair treatments in one session to get faster results, such as a microdermabrasion and a chemical peel, or a dermaplaning and a microcurrent treatment.

Offer a treatment plan that is comprehensive and includes the professional sessions as well as the home skincare that they will need to get their skin to a healthy condition. Set your client's expectations. For a client who has aging skin, you can perform treatments and recommend skincare products that build collagen and improve the skin's overall health.

Microdermabrasion/Infused Microdermabrasion

Nordic skin responds well to microdermabrasion and is an excellent option to remove layers of dry skin. By removing layers of the stratum corneum, other treatments can work more effectively and skincare products can penetrate easier. Be mindful of your client's thinner skin and don't be too aggressive until you know your client's skin can tolerate it.

Adding hydration with an infusion treatment is an excellent way to maintain homeostasis with TEWL.

Microdermabrasion is not a treatment for someone with rosacea. The suction and aggressive exfoliation can increase telangiectasias and even cause bruising.

Chemical Peels

Clients with Fitzpatrick skin type 1 or 2 should respond well to chemical peels. Chemical peels are excellent options for treating concerns with anti-aging; however, verify that your client doesn't have a sensitivity to the peel ingredients. Although a series of chemical peels can build collagen, they are not the option for addressing skin laxity.

You may not have to condition your Nordic client's skin the same way you would with darker Fitzpatrick skin types by increasing chemical peel acid strengths and percentages. Your client should be able to tolerate a glycolic peel or more aggressive peel with little risk of complications. Nordic skin can tolerate "cocktailed" peels that contain a combination of ingredients, like glycolic, TCA, resorcinol, phenol, and tretinoin. Your client should be able to tolerate a heat sensation that reaches a level 8.

You may condition the skin during the peel series with the number of passes you apply to the skin.

Facial Devices

Nordic skin will respond favorably to radio frequency for skin tightening. Fractional radio frequency with microneedling is a more aggressive treatment that will benefit skin texture including fine lines and skin laxity. Microneedling has even been proven to strengthen the dermis and reduce the amount of erythema in rosacea clients.[11] Electrical devices like ultrasonic spatula (for exfoliation and infusion), high frequency, and microcurrent are tools that can be used with confidence on this skin type. With any treatment, a series of sessions will condition the skin and give a better outcome.

Due to the ineffectiveness of laser hair removal on very light hair, dermaplaning or waxing may be the best option for your Nordic client.

Lasers and IPL

Fractional laser treatments are ideal for Nordic clients seeking immediate results. IPL or laser skin rejuvenation show visible results within a short time of beginning a series. Laser resurfacing treatments for overall skin improvements can also be done with the expectation of good results.

Your Nordic client may not have hair that's dark enough for effective laser hair removal sessions, as there may not be enough melanin in the hair follicle to absorb the laser and kill the follicle.

Combination Treatments

Combination treatments are a strong option for your client's plan of care. Nordic skin, although thin, has resilience and can tolerate the effects of two different approaches to the skin in one treatment session. There is little risk of post-inflammatory hyperpigmentation (PIH), although with very thin and vascular skin, your client may experience post-inflammatory hypervascularity or extended skin erythema that will eventually resolve. A calming mask or LED light therapy at the end of your treatment will be helpful.

Home Skincare Recommendations

A solid skin analysis is the key to getting your client on a successful home skincare regimen. Using gentle ingredients when you are first working with your client will help them build trust in your skills. Take time in the consultation to explain the reasons behind your treatment plan and your commitment to reduce the risk of impaired barrier function response. You can steadily add more potent ingredients as you become familiar with your client's skin's reactions and tolerance levels.

Harsh ingredients that compromise barrier function are ones to stay away from if your client has issues with TEWL skin sensitivity.

When creating a home care plan, you can confidently move forward with antioxidants and growth factors to build collagen and improve the thickness of the dermis. Moisturizers with ingredients that are low on the comedogenic scale are great options.

BB creams that are multifunctional may be good options for your Nordic client who is looking for a "less is more" skincare regimen.

Conclusion

People from Nordic countries and Ireland need solid skincare professionals to guide their treatment plan and achieve healthier skin. By being mindful of the structural changes as well as skin diseases and disorders that are more common to this skin type, you will elevate your level of professional expertise.

You'll increase word-of-mouth referrals and develop a loyal client base by demonstrating your understanding of the unique characteristics of Nordic skin.

NOTES

1. Sharrie Williams, "Red Hot Lipstick and Maybelline Eyes, Personified 1950's Hollywood Stars and Still Does Today," The Maybelline Story, January 30, 2014, accessed March 28, 2019, https://www.maybellinebook.com/2014/01/maybellines-new-color-elixir-lip-gloss.html.

2. Saioa López, "Skin Color: An Example of Adaptation to the Environment," Sruk, January 12, 2017, accessed March 28, 2019, https://sruk.org.uk/skin-color-an-example-of-adaptation-to-the-environment/.

3. Rasmus Kragh Jakobsen, "Scandinavians Are the Earliest Europeans," *ScienceNordic*, November 19, 2014, accessed March 28, 2019, http://sciencenordic.com/scandinavians-are-earliest-europeans.

4. Allison Van Dusen, "World's Skin Cancer Hot Spots," *Forbes*, July 28, 2008, accessed March 28, 2019, https://www.forbes.com/2008/07/28/skin-cancer-hotspots-forbeslife-cx_avd_0728health.html#29fe1c891424.

5. "Sarcoidosis," American Academy of Dermatology, accessed March 28, 2019, https://www.aad.org/public/diseases/bumps-and-growths/sarcoidosis#causes.

6. Marianne Baksjøberg, "Learning about Allergies from Skin Disease," *ScienceNordic*, February 20, 2012, accessed March 28, 2019, http://sciencenordic.com/learning-about-allergies-skin-disease.

7. Lynn Drake, ed. "New Evidence Shows Rosacea May Be Linked to Heredity," *Rosacea Review*, (Fall 1996), https://www.rosacea.org/rosacea-review/1996/fall/new-evidence-shows-rosacea-may-be-linked-to-heredity.

8. "Viking Inventions," The Vikings History, accessed March 28, 2019, https://thevikingshistory.weebly.com/viking-inventions.html.

9. Stina Backer, "Nordic Delights: The Scandinavian Diet Is among the Healthiest and Most Delicious in the World." *The Independent*, March 26, 2009, accessed March 28, 2019, https://www.independent.co.uk/life-style/food-and-drink/features/nordic-delights-the-scandinavian-diet-is-among-the-healthiest-and-most-delicious-in-the-world-1654155.html.

10. Erin Jahns, "What Scandinavian Women Know About Glowing Skin (That You Don't)," *Byrdie*, February 9, 2018, accessed March 28, 2019, https://www.byrdie.com/scandinavian-beauty-secrets.

11. "Microneedling Opens Door for Rosacea Relief," Skin Inc. April 24, 2017, accessed March 28, 2019, https://www.skininc.com/spabusiness/medicalesthetics/Microneedling-Opens-Door-for-Rosacea-Relief-416725213.html.

Fig 6.2. Sharrie Williams, "Maybelline and the teenage market, Post WW II, USA," The Maybelline Story, June 28, 2011, accessed March 28, 2019, https://www.maybellinebook.com/2011/06/maybelline-and-teenage-market-post-ww.html.

Fig 6.4. George Chaplin, "Geographic Distribution of Environmental Factors Influencing Human Skin Coloration," *American Journal of Physical Anthropology* 125, no 3, (Nov 2004): 292-302, fig 3, fig updated 2007, https://doi.org/10.1002/ajpa.10263.

Fig 6.6. Gabriel Hildebrand, *Comb Bone/antler*, July 4, 2013, photograph, The Swedish History Museum, Flickr, https://www.flickr.com/photos/historiska/13622352435/in/photostream/.

Gabriel Hildebrand, *Comb Bone/antler*, July 4, 2013, photograph, The Swedish History Museum, Flickr, https://https://www.flickr.com/photos/historiska/13622369573/in/photostream/.

https://creativecommons.org/licenses/by/2.0/legalcode

Fig 6.7. *Tweezers*, February 25, 2011, photograph, The Swedish History Museum, Flickr, https://www.flickr.com/photos/historiska/6875889819/in/album-72157629316810373/.

https://creativecommons.org/licenses/by/2.0/legalcode

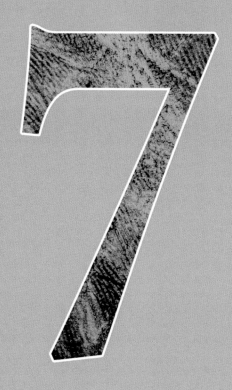

7
MULTI-ETHNIC SKIN

MULTI-ETHNIC SKIN

We've looked at the specifics involved in treating distinct ethnicities. Now we are going to delve into the processes regarding the consultation and developing a treatment plan when you have a multi-ethnic client (fig 7.1). As the United States becomes increasingly blended, developing the best treatment plan for your client will depend even more on your skills with interviewing and performing skin analysis. Your client's skin color may not reflect their mixed heritage, and you could experience adverse events, like scarring, burns, blisters, hyper- and hypo-pigmentation if you do not perform a proper analysis.

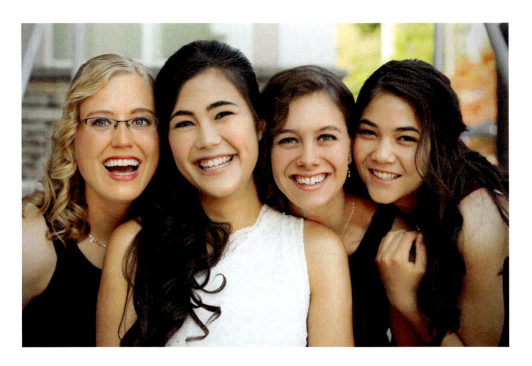

Your client's skin color may not reflect their mixed heritage. Photo source: Jaren Wicklund/stock.adobe.com.
(7.1)

Client Information and Health History

In order to provide you with the most appropriate treatment, we need you to complete the following questionnaire. All information is confidential.

Client Name: _____   Date of Birth: _____

Email Address: _____   Phone Number: _____

Home Address: _____

How were you referred to us? _____ Occupation: _____

Which of the following best describes your skin type? (Please circle one number)

- I. Fair-always burns, never tans
- II. Light skin tones-can burn, sometimes tans
- III. Medium to olive skin tones, tans easily
- IV. Medium to dark skin tones
- V. Brown, moderately pigmented skin
- VI. Black skin

Medical History

Are you currently under the care of a medical professional for any reason?   ☐ Yes   ☐ No

If yes, for what _____

SEX	☐ Male	☐ Female	☐ Other	Preferred Pronoun?
HISTORY		YES	NO	DATE/LIST/COMMENTS
LIST ALL MEDICATIONS, SUPPLEMENTS AND/OR VITAMINS				
Accutane				
Antibiotics				
Birth Control Pills				
Hormones				
Aspirin, Ibuprofen use				
Retin A, Tretinoin				
Metro Gel, Metro Cream				
Antidepressants				
LIST ALLERGIES				
Sun Reactions				
Medication Allergies				
Food Allergies				
Aspirin Allergy				
Latex Allergy				
Lidocaine Allergy				
Hydrocortisone Allergy				
Hydroquinone Allergy				
Dairy Intolerance				
Do you eat a healthy diet?		When did you last eat processed/fast food?		
Water Intake Daily		Alcohol Intake Daily		Caffeine

Callouts:
- You need age related information to formulate a good plan. Skin changes with age.
- This could influence your treatment choice. Do they work outside? Are they under HEV lightning? Think about how their job could affect their skin.
- This helps you understand how your client views their skin. You will still need to perform a skin analysis and determine skin type.
- Underlying medical conditions can influence the skin and affect healing.
- Helps you determine your client's gender identity and creates trust in how they want to be addressed.
- Medications influence the skin and certain medications are contraindicated for some treatments.
- You need to know allergies so you don't apply products that could cause an adverse reaction.
- Your client's eating habits are reflected in their skin.

The client information and medical history form contains vital pieces of information that you'll need to develop an appropriate treatment plan. Take your time reviewing it in the consultation. Graphic source: Sarah Jensen.

(7.2)

Your client may look like a Fitzpatrick skin type 2, but after investigation, you may find that your client has a grandmother who is Asian. Your knowledge and intuition ought to tell you that your client's skin will respond like a Fitzpatrick skin type 4.

Some practitioners are concerned that asking clients about their ethnicity will make it seem like they are discriminating or prejudiced. Investigating your client's ancestry is not racist if the purpose is to accurately treat skin. It's the responsibility of an ethical practitioner and will save you hours of tears and headache when you

HISTORY		
Diabetes		
Smoking History		
Cold Sores, Herpes		
Bleeding Disorders		
Autoimmune, HIV		
Pregnant, Planning to be		
Pacemaker		
Implants of any kind - dental, breast		
Migraine Headaches		
Glaucoma		
Cancer		
Arthritis		
Hepatitis		
Thyroid Imbalance		
Seizure Disorder		
Active Infection		
Radiation in last 3 months		
SKIN CONDITIONS		
Acne		
Melasma		
Tattoos, Perm. Makeup, Microblading		
Vitiligo		
Keloid Scarring		
Skin/Laser Treatments at another office	If so, when?	Results
Botox	If so, when?	Results
Fillers	If so, when?	Results
Hair Removal	If so, when?	Results
Chemical Peels	If so, when?	Results
Sun exposure/tanning bed in last week? Self Tanner?	If so, when?	Results
HOME SKIN CARE		

Annotations:
- Diabetes could influence healing times.
- Smoking can impair wound healing and getting oxygen to tissues.
- Pregnancy and lactation is a contraindication for most treatments.
- Pacemaker can be a contraindication for a radio frequency or microcurrent treatment.
- Seizures are contraindicated for LED.
- Laser treatments can't be performed over tattoos, permanent makeup or microblading.
- Treatments at another office need to be investigated further.
- Tanning is a contraindication as well as self tanner for some treatments.

How would you describe your skin condition: ☐ Oily ☐ Dry ☐ Sensitive ☐ Normal ☐ Combination

☐ I'm concerned about fine lines around my eyes.
☐ I'm concerned about pigmentation or age spots.
☐ I'm concerned about skin laxity and sagging.
☐ I'm concerned about the lines around my mouth.
☐ I'm concerned about broken capillaries on my face or spider veins on my legs.

I certify that the preceding medical, personal and skin history statements are true and correct. I am aware that it is my responsibility to inform the technician of my current medical and health conditions and to update this information at subsequent visits. A current history is essential for the provider to execute appropriate treatment procedures. I have signed the consent form for this procedure. I have the opportunity to ask questions prior to the treatment.

_____ _____
Signature Client   Date

_____ _____
Reviewed by Skincare Professional   Date

take the time to perform a thorough consultation. By explaining that your intent is to find a treatment that's customized perfectly to the client's skincare needs and different skin types respond differently to treatments even with the same color, you will educate your client as well as build confidence and trust.

Each of the questions on the client health and history form is intended to give you an insight into your client's individual skin needs (fig 7.2). If your client has marked anything on the form, verbally confirm the details and get more information. Investigate further with questions so you have a clear understanding of your client's lifestyle, diet, water intake, activities, home skincare, and more.

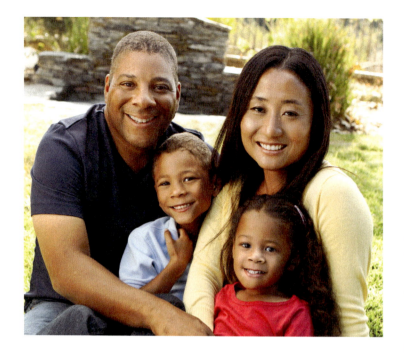

Multi-ethnic families are becoming more prevalent. In the 2000 census over 6.8 million Americans selected that they identified with two or more races.[1] Photo source: pixelheadphoto digitalskillet/ Shutterstock.com.
(7.3)

What Are the Characteristics

Clients who are multi-ethnic need you to be aware of all of the ethnicities in their heritage. You can have a client who is ¼ Asian, ¼ South Asian, ¼ Nordic, and ¼ Latinx, depending on the heritage of their parents and grandparents (fig 7.3). You will need to factor in your knowledge of these ethnicities before creating a plan of care that will achieve results but not be too aggressive so your client develops post-inflammatory hyperpigmentation (PIH) or another form of hyperpigmentation.

Many different ethnicities have similar skin structure issues. Concerns about hyperpigmentation, trans epidermal water loss (TEWL), and barrier function are common concerns with darker Fitzpatrick skin types regardless of ethnicity.

Diseases and Disorders

Be mindful of the diseases and disorders that more commonly afflict certain ethnicities. Question your multi-ethnic Asian clients on lactose tolerance, melasma, and acne. Make sure you are examining the skin for periorbital hyperpigmentation, melasma, and acne with multi-ethnic South Asian clients. Determine whether or not diabetes is a concern with multi-ethnic Latinx clients. Polycystic ovary syndrome (PCOS), fibroids and the accompanying symptoms manifest on the skin with Black clients. With multi-ethnic Nordic skin, look for signs of rosacea and be alert to unusual pigmentation that could mean skin cancer. With a transgender client, you'll want to pay close attention to hormones, other medications, and the possibility of an autoimmune disorder. If your client is Black and Asian, you'll have to consider the skin characteristics and common disorders of a client who is Black and Asian.

Cultural and Dietary Practices

America is a melting pot of cultures so your multi-ethnic client may have a variety of cultures integrated into their lifestyle (fig 7.4). They may have adopted cultures from the native country of their family or blended cultures and traditions from several ethnicities and backgrounds.

Once you've started your treatment plan, you may have to investigate further into your client's lifestyle if you are not seeing the anticipated results. Clients may be embarrassed to tell you about their diet or skincare practices, particularly if they are new to seeing a skincare professional.

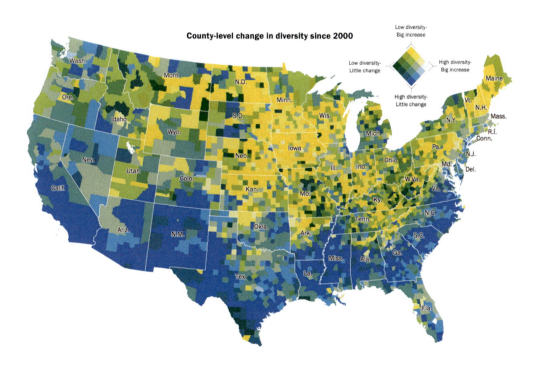

A 2016 study by the Washington Post shows how the United States is becoming increasingly diverse. With rapid change occurring in the Midwest, a place that had very little diversity prior to 2000 but that now is changing to a multicultural mix. Map source: Keating and Karklis, "The increasingly diverse," *The Washington Post*.
(7.4)

The Consultation

The consultation is a key component to establishing trust with your client (fig 7.5). You can find out your client's goals for skin improvements and also set the appropriate expectations for treatments. Professional skincare is a rewarding process, and it's worth being intentional in your conversation with your client and in your physical exam of the skin.

Accurately document findings and details about your client's diet, lifestyle, sleep habits, stress levels, etc. It's a good reference for future treatment plans and goals as well as a protection in a liability situation.

When you have a client who wants treatment to improve acne, here are some points and considerations to include in your consultation:

- Diet, including dairy and processed food intake. These can contribute to breakouts.
- Alcohol intake. Alcohol is dehydrating and can cause retention keratosis.
- Water intake. Hydration affects the entire body, and dehydration will create dryness that will influence comedone production.
- Does your client wear a cap regularly? How often is it cleaned? Unclean ball caps can cause forehead breakouts. Adolescents that play school sports may have increased breakouts from helmet chin straps as well.

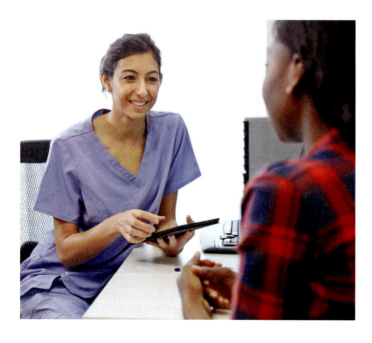

Your client will appreciate the time you take for a thorough consultation. It builds trust and rapport. Photo source: Monkey Business/stock.adobe.com.
(7.5)

- Does your client participate in sports or exercise? Cleaning the face to remove sweat as soon as possible will help.
- How often does your client change their pillowcase? Dirt and sebum sticks to the pillowcase and can influence breakouts.
- Does your client wear a silk scarf at night? How often is it cleaned? Silk scarves can increase the incidence of hairline acne.
- Hormones and medications. Medications that are intended to balance hormones and help with PCOS are often estrogen influencers that can cause acne.
- Fabric softeners have oils and fragrances that can affect the skin when in contact with the skin.
- How often your male clients replace their razor is significant. Razor blades can harbor bacteria.
- Cell phone screens can spread bacteria if the screen is not cleaned regularly.
- Does your client use a Clarisonic or other type of cleansing device? Is it sanitized regularly?
- If your client's breakouts are predominantly perioral, hormones may be the cause, but consider the type of toothpaste your client is using. An allergy can spark a breakout of dermatitis that will look like acne.
- If your client has pigmentation issues, you need a thorough physical exam to determine if it is melasma, sun damage, or some other type of hyperpigmentation. With melasma, look for a solid symmetrical pattern rather than pigmented lesions.

Here are a few questions to delve deeper into your client's pigmentation:

- Does the pigmentation seem to come and go depending on the weather?
- Does your client use light therapy for Seasonal Affective Disorder (SAD)? Wavelength around 300 nm can cause pigmentation.
- Does your client have a family history of PCOS? Have they been diagnosed with a hormonal disorder?
- Does your client wear SPF sunscreen religiously? Do they reapply every 90 minutes?
- Is your client on birth control pills or taking hormonal supplements for menopause transitioning?
- Does your client eat a lot of soy based foods? Soy contains hormones.
- Is your client a hot-yoga fan? Or other heat-based activities?

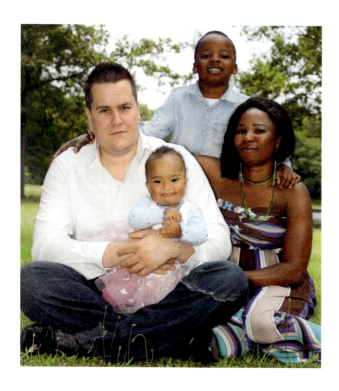

Lifestyle issues, like being a busy parent, should be a consideration in the consultation. Photo source: Frank Kaufmann/stock.adobe.com.

(7.6)

Clients with rosacea will need a consultation that includes conversations about the following:

- Does your client have Nordic heritage?
- Does your client have a family history of facial redness, even if there is no diagnosis of rosacea?
- Is your client experiencing itching, burning and swelling? Rosacea sufferers experience varying degrees of itching and burning sensations and may experience edema due vascular congestion.
- Is your client experiencing dry and flaky skin despite experiencing what seems like acne breakouts? Rosacea clients can have both dry or oily skin but dry flaking is more common.
- Does your client also experience seborrheic dermatitis? A high percentage of rosacea clients also experience patches of seborrheic dermatitis between the brows or on the scalp.
- Is your client able to identify specific triggers that increase redness, flushing and irritation such as sun exposure, emotional stress, hot or cold weather, alcohol, spicy foods, heavy exercise, hot baths or showers, and some skincare products?

With any client, you need to ask about budget and commitment (fig 7.6). If your client is on a limited budget, focus on home care first. Map out a plan to add the appropriate skincare products and then add in the professional treatments. Even if your client has an unlimited budget, add skincare slowly. If your client has an adverse reaction, it will be much easier to determine the reason if you are having to evaluate one or two products, versus a full home care regimen of seven or eight products.

You must also talk to your client seriously about their skincare commitment. For a client who has a simplistic beauty regimens, wears little makeup, and never uses moisturizer or SPF protection, it's unrealistic to expect them to begin a twice-daily regimen of multiple products. The client who is a product junkie at Sephora, on the other hand, will appreciate your guidance in setting them up with a full regimen of skincare that will be tailored specifically for their skin.

In order to find a root cause of your client's skin issue and find the best solution, it is important to ask many questions and not assume things about your client. When you take the time to perform a thorough consultation, you are building a relationship with your client and demonstrating your skills as a professional.

The Treatment Plan

Your consultation will guide you to the best treatment plan for your multi-ethnic client. Offer a treatment plan that is comprehensive and includes professional sessions as well as home skincare that will get their skin to a healthy condition. Because of the risks of PIH with multi-ethnic skin, you will need to condition your client's skin and build up a tolerance to progressively stronger ingredients and treatments.[2] All darker skin types battle PIH after a skin injury or inflammation, so recognizing and treating PIH as soon as it is identified will help lessen the severity and recovery time.

Understand that aggressive treatments can affect the acid-mantle balance and create a barrier function problem. Inform your clients who are anxious for immediate results that slow and steady, progressive rather than aggressive, is the safest plan to help your multi-ethnic clients.

Consider all of the tools in your aesthetic toolbox and approach your client's skin with a combination of modalities. Once your client's skin is conditioned with home skincare and single treatment sessions, you can consider combination treatments performed at the same appointment session. Your client will benefit from combination treatments that approach the skin problem from different angles. Dermaplaning with a chemical peel or fractional collagen induction with skin tightening radio frequency are two of the options that may be beneficial combination treatments for your clients.

See your client two weeks after the initial consultation. At the two-week appointment, check in and make sure your client is being cooperative with home skincare and begin a series of office treatments. An enzyme exfoliation or a superficial chemical peel is a great first treatment option. It will add some radiance by removing some dull stratum corneum buildup. See your client in two-to-three-week intervals until trust is established. Take photos at each appointment so you and your client can review the progress. Reevaluate your treatment plan based on your client's feedback and the photos.

Home Skincare Recommendations

When first working with your client, use gentle ingredients rather than harsh ones that compromise barrier function. Explaining your reasons and your commitment to reducing the risk of negative reactions will help build trust in your skills.

Start your client on a gentle cleanser and pH-balancing toner. Address any kind of pigmentation with a plant/fungus-based melanin inhibitor. You can recommend hydroquinone for short-term use by titrating the strength from 2% to 4% and then back down. Return to a non-hydroquinone product for their daily regimen. In times of hot weather, or if hormones are fluctuating, you may need to resume a short-term use of hydroquinone to bring the melanin production under control. Make your recommendation for a moisturizer based on your skin assessment.

Multi-ethnic skin responds well to epidermal growth factors and antioxidant serums to nourish the skin and build collagen.

When working with the acneic client, consider adding salicylic acid, benzoyl peroxide, and retinoic acids in small percentages. You will see improvements but the skin will develop a tolerance, so you'll need to increase the strength to initiate continued changes in the skin.

Start slowly and incorporate professional treatments such as LED blue-light therapy to control the *p. acnes* bacteria.

Conclusion

"Multi-ethnic skin" refers to a variety of skin colors, nationalities, and geographical influences. Approach the multi-ethnic client with confidence in your ability to perform a comprehensive skin consultation and analysis. Apply your understanding of how diseases and disorders are presented, the unique characteristics, as well as your awareness of cultural practices, lifestyle choices, and dietary indications that will affect the skin. Combine your knowledge of different ethnicities to make the best plan of care for your client.

Elevate your profession by being knowledgeable about multi-ethnic skin. Your ability to effectively care for multi-ethnic skin will determine your success as a skincare professional.

NOTES

1. "Multiracial Profile," CensusScope, accessed September 7, 2020, http://www.censusscope.org/us/chart_multi.html.

2. Stephanie Nouveau, Divya Agrawal, Malavika Kohli, Francoise Bernerd, Namita Misra, and Chitra Shivanand Nayak, "Skin Hyperpigmentation in Indian Population: Insights and Best Practice," *Indian Journal of Dermatology* 61, no. 5 (September/October 2016): 487-95, doi:10.4103/0019-5154.190103.

Fig 7.4. Dan Keating and Laris Karklis, "The increasingly diverse United States of America," *The Washington Post*, Nov 25, 2016, accessed April 17, 2019, https://www.washingtonpost.com/graphics/national/how-diverse-is-america/.

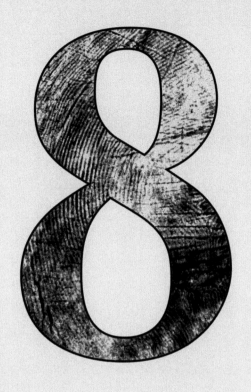

TRANSGENDER CLIENTS

TRANSGENDER CLIENTS

Transgender clients will have particular needs you may not be prepared for. Educating yourself on how to treat transgender clients will make you more comfortable in your approach and communications as well as lessen the chance that you will appear insensitive or even offend your client unintentionally.

There may be significant psychological, socio-economic, familial and regulatory issues that will require your awareness. Your transgender client may have concerns about discrimination, so your willingness to assure them your acceptance of their gender identity is going to make a big difference in building a trusting long-term relationship (fig 8.1).

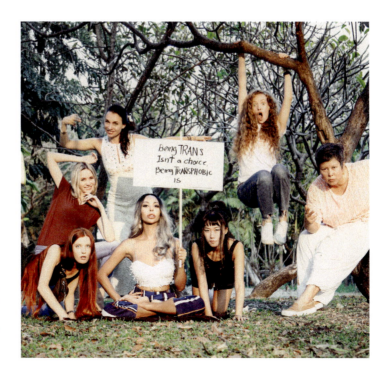

Remember that being trans isn't a choice, but that being transphobic is. Open-minded kindness and acceptance is important when working with **transgender clients.** Photo Source: Radharani/Shutterstock.com.

(8.1)

Let's talk about some overall education on transgender and then dive into specifics with skin and skincare.[1]

Transgender is a broad term that is used to describe someone whose gender identity or gender expression doesn't conform with their assigned sex.

Gender identity refers to a person's sense that they are male, female, or another gender (fig 8.2).

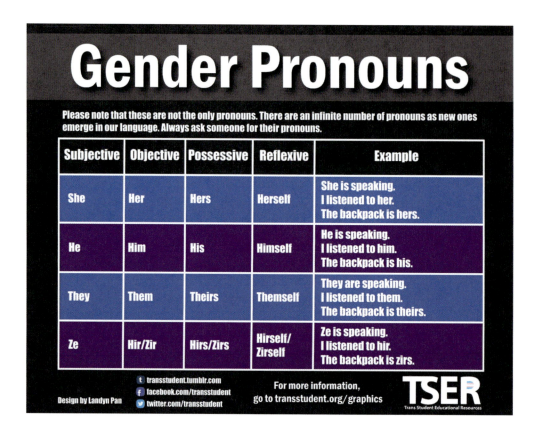

It is important to ask clients for their preferred pronoun in your initial consultation. Asking and correctly using a client's pronouns is a basic way that you can show respect for their gender identity. Graphic source: Pan, *Gender Pronouns*, TSER.
(8.2)

Gender expression is how a person communicates their gender vocally as well as with clothing, behavior, body art, hairstyles, and more.

Sex refers to the assignment of male or female at birth. The assignment is based on chromosomes, hormones, and physical anatomy. Gender norms refer to societal culture and influence that determines what is appropriate behavior, dress, speech, professions, and more for each sex.

Some people choose to undergo hormone therapy, surgery and more to alter their bodies to reflect their gender identity. Transsexual refers to someone whose gender identity is different from their birth sex assignment and has changed or wishes to change their sex through medical intervention. However, the transgender community considers the term transsexual contentious because it was historically used to describe transgender individuals as mentally ill. Hence, the negative association. Avoid using transsexual to describe someone unless they use it to refer to themselves.[2]

Crossdressing is a form of gender expression where a person wears clothing that is typically worn by the opposite sex. A person who enjoys crossdressing does not necessarily identify as transgender.

Gender non-conforming describes some people whose gender expression is different from conventional expectations of masculinity and femininity. Not all gender non-conforming people identify as transgender, and not all transgender people are gender non-conforming. Many people have gender expressions that are not entirely conventional— this fact alone does not make them transgender. Many transgender men and women have gender expressions that are conventionally masculine or feminine.[3]

Transitioning from one gender to another is a complicated process. Most transgender people start communicating their decisions in settings where they feel safe. Changes are made gradually. Common changes include adopting the clothing and grooming of the gender they identify with as well as a name change. For gender reassignment, often times called gender affirmation surgery, a medical professional will guide the person through medication and hormone therapy.

Jeanne is a trans woman in her fifties. For her fortieth birthday milestone, she finally decided to give herself permission to be who she was. Jeanne, formerly John, was raised in a loving family but always struggled to meet her parents' expectations to be a rough and tumble boy. She was happy playing "house" with her sisters and never adopted the cocky adolescent male attitude. She always, had a vague feeling that she didn't fit in with the neighborhood boys. She had several girlfriends in high school but was not particularly interested in physical intimacy. She was ashamed to admit that she was attracted to several male friends. Once Jeanne left home for college, she began to open herself up to the idea that she was gay. After researching everything she could, taking gender studies and classes on human sexuality, she decided to accept that she was transsexual. Her

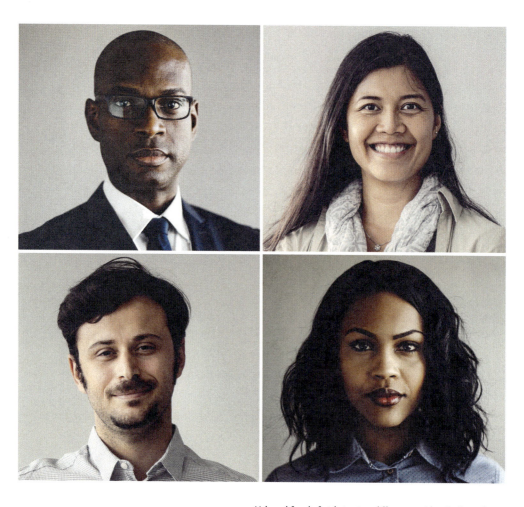

Male and female facial structure differences evident in these photos.
Photo source: Flamingo Images & sebra/stock.adobe.com, edited by Sarah Jensen.
(8.3)

gender identity was female but her physical anatomy was male. Society's bias against homosexuality at the time kept her from revealing her identity. For years, she enjoyed private time when she could paint her nails, try on different hair styles with wigs, experiment with different makeup looks, and wear the style of clothing that reflected her view of herself, but she felt like a loner. The gay pride parade and other local support systems began to emerge, and when Jeanne was close to her fortieth birthday, she took two weeks off work. When she returned from her vacation, she returned openly as Jeanne. Coworkers were surprised, but most quickly came to accept her. She was open to discussions and was asked to lead a diversity task force at her tech company. She began counseling for Gender Confirmation surgery and looks forward to what is in store for her future.

What You Need to Know

Some transgender clients decide to undergo medical intervention, while others opt against it. It's an extremely personal and costly decision.

Female and male faces have some aesthetic differences (fig 8.3).[4] The female face has a flatter forehead, more open eyes with arched eyebrows, prominent cheekbones, and full lips. The male face has a rounder forehead, smaller eyes with flattened eyebrows, and a more angular jawline.

There are skin structure differences as well.[5]

- Men have larger sebaceous glands and larger pores and produce more sebum.
- Female skin is smoother and finer because the stratum corneum is thinner than in male skin. Men lose subcutaneous fat faster than females, which causes deeper facial wrinkling with aging.
- Male skin is approximately 25% thicker than female skin. A woman's skin thickness remains constant until menopause, when hormones shift significantly. Male skin gradually thins with age.
- Collagen fibers are packed more densely in men's skin. Women may show signs of aging earlier because their skin structure doesn't have as much collagen support.
- Male facial hair is thicker, denser and follicles are deeper. Shaving is a form of exfoliation but frequent shaving may create microscopic injuries to the skin and weaken barrier function.

Diseases and Disorders

There are few studies documenting disease and disorder issues with the transgender population, but there are some considerations for you to be aware of.

- The high cost of hormone therapy, disrespectful or ignorant treatment by medical professionals, and restricted access to healthcare has created a black market for the use of illegal or questionably legal substances being ingested or injected. In a study in San Francisco with 314 transgender women, 49% were taking hormones not prescribed by a medical professional.[6] Cosmetic injectables are also a black market product that your client may be using to acquire facial features that appear more like the gender they identify with. Your transgender client may have infections or granulomas from both of these types of treatments. Granulomas are hard cyst-like lumps that form when the body's immune system reacts to a foreign substance by creating a thick shell around it. Granulomas and infections should be treated by a medical professional.

- One study indicates transgender women have a higher incidence of the autoimmune disease lupus erythematosus.[7] It is believed this is due to long-term estrogen therapy. Lupus erythematosus has severe onset and can affect cardiovascular as well as kidney functions.[8]

- A study in 2013 from The Centers for Disease Control and Prevention (CDC) reports that transgender women have a higher incidence of HIV and sexually transmitted infections. The CDC suggests certain risk factors directly tied to transphobia and the marginalization that transgender people face that may contribute to such high infection rates. These risk factors include "higher rates of drug and alcohol abuse, sex work, incarceration, homelessness, attempted suicide, unemployment, lack of familial support, violence, stigma and discrimination, limited health care access, and negative health care encounters."[9]

- HIV has skin-related symptoms such as fungal infections, seborrheic dermatitis, eczema, and pruritic papules.[10] When creating a treatment plan, you would take an active infection into consideration and most treatments would not be appropriate. Eczema and pruritic papules could lead to barrier function compromise, another consideration during the consultation and treatment plan process.

- Among transgender men in transition, testosterone is used to suppress female sex characteristics. The drug is usually given via a weekly injection, although there is a longer lasting drug that is used off-label and given every twelve weeks. It is important for the medical professional to be aware of the possibility of osteoporosis. Additionally, medical professionals will be regularly checking lipid blood levels, indicating cholesterol levels, and hematocrit blood levels checking for red blood cell activity and dehydration. Weekly injections may continue for six months to a year and then the client will transition to implanted testosterone pellets. The pellets are inserted under the skin into a fatty area of the body like the hip or buttocks. About 1/3 of the pellet dose is absorbed in the first month. Twenty five percent is absorbed in the second month and one sixth during the third month. Most clients require reimplantation of pellets every three to four months.

- Within three months of starting hormone therapy, your client will have increased facial and body hair, increased acne, changes in fat distribution, libido and muscle mass. Menstruation will have stopped. The voice will begin to deepen, the vagina walls will thin and the clitoris will enlarge. Male pattern hair loss is also evident.

- Breast reduction is usually the first surgery that your transgender male client will undergo during transition.[11] There are a number of different surgical techniques that include repositioning the nipple and removing the breast tissue depending on the size of the client's breasts and skin health. Scarring will occur due to breast reduction surgery.

- Transgender female clients transitioning will undergo hormone therapy that will change fat distribution, reduce male pattern hair growth and increased breast size and experience loss of erectile function. Estrogen is the main hormone but must be balanced with other testosterone inhibiting medications in order to work effectively. Spironolactone is a common medication prescribed to suppress testosterone. Spironolactone use has a side effect of high blood potassium levels and your client may experience weakness, irregular heartbeat, nausea and muscle cramps. Initial hormone therapy can take eighteen to twenty-four months.

- Sex organ anatomical differences due to hormones and surgery may be a consideration for you as well if you are performing intimate waxing or laser hair removal.

Your open-minded kindness and acceptance is important when making the best for your transgender clients.

The Consultation

You may not even know your client is transgender, as you cannot tell someone is transgender by just looking at them. Adapting your client intake and history form to ask all clients to indicate their gender identity, may give you an indication that your client is transgender if they do not disclose it. Asking which pronoun your client prefers will also send an important message. If your client is transitioning from male to female and prefers to be referenced as "she," it is critical that you remember to use that pronoun. Referring to your client's significant other as "spouse" or "partner" is also more appropriate than using "boyfriend/girlfriend" or "husband/wife."

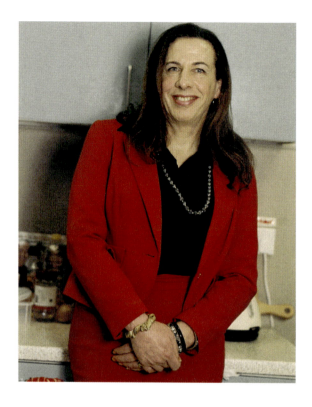

You'll need to consider the interplay of many factors when developing your treatment. Photo source: Bex Day/stock.adobe.com.
(8.4)

Another indication that your client is transgender are the medications your client is taking. Hormones are a good example. Women may be taking hormone supplements or replacements for any number of reasons: hormonal imbalances, to ease the symptoms of menopause, or possibly because your client is transitioning. "I see you're taking hormones. Can you tell me more about that. The reason I'm asking is hormones can affect skin and treatment. And we want to avoid side effects." is a good conversation starter. It is important to explain to your client why you're asking these questions to make your client comfortable and to build trust. Hormones have a significant effect on the skin and can determine which treatment option will result in the best outcome for your client. Hormone supplements may be the contributing cause of your client's acne, for example. Knowing that information will help you set the right expectations for treatment.

Be prepared for modesty when treating your transgender client. They may have already endured negative comments on their journey and need to be in a safe place when receiving your services. A client coming in for hair removal services as they are transitioning needs your respect. Gender reassignment surgery may not be complete, so giving your client privacy while undressing to don a spa gown or robe is important. Appropriate draping will help relieve any anxiety.

Respecting your client's privacy by not discussing their treatments or your experience with them to other clients or even other staff is your professional responsibility. It will create a strong level of trust with your client.

Give yourself enough time to thoroughly consider all issues affecting your client's skin (fig 8.4). In addition to the differences in multi-ethnic skin, you are going to have to consider your client's birth gender as well as determine the hormonal influences of medication.

You need to ask questions that investigate your client's ethnicity, Fitzpatrick skin type, and lifestyle and dietary choices, as well as review your client's medical history. Also, a review of your client's medications is essential. In addition to hormone supplements, your client may be taking medication for other medical issues that you need to be aware of. Research the side effects of their medication to ensure no treatment you recommend is contraindicated. A conference with your client's medical provider should also be considered as a more holistic effort at addressing your client's concerns.

Set the expectation that your client will need a series of skincare treatments as well as a regimen of home skincare in the same manner that you would with any other client.

Get photos of your client's skin as a baseline for comparison. Get photos in a front view, and side views.

The Treatment Plan

As your transgender client may not have a beauty culture established, they may need education on skincare and treatment. You can help provide that foundation.

Your transgender female client may initially come to you for hair removal services. Once you have established a level of trust, you may be able to introduce her to other services for pore refinement, texture changes, fine lines, and more that will soften and feminize her features.

Your transgender male client may be wanting acne breakout relief. He'll need assurance that your acne treatments will be treating the symptoms but curing the acne will not be possible during hormone therapy. He'll see some skin relief as hormone levels become stable, but ongoing treatment is recommended.

You'll need to consider the interplay of many factors when developing your plan. Your client's gender at birth, along with their heritage and ethnic background, is as much a consideration as the hormones they are taking to support their gender identification and medications for other medical issues. Be sure to update your client's medical history at every visit, including medications.

Your consultation will guide you to the best treatment plan for your client, but you will need to remain flexible, so your client will have confidence in your skills when you make changes.

Microdermabrasion/Infused Microdermabrasion

Microdermabrasion is a great choice for removing dead skin cells from the stratum corneum and can be effective in helping to reduce keratinization buildup with transgender male clients. It is not the recommended treatment for feminizing your transgender female clients. The results aren't intended to soften features.

Chemical Peels

Chemical peels may be an option for hyperpigmentation, but they can also work to reduce the appearance of pore size and refine texture. This may help to create a softer look for your transgender female clients, but if your client also has multi-ethnic skin, you will need to titrate the chemical peel percentage and build your client's ability to tolerate the acids in the same way as any other multi-ethnic client so you are not risking post-inflammatory hyperpigmentation (PIH) or other adverse effects.

A chemical peel series may also improve acne breakouts for transgender male clients.

As with any client, make sure there are no contraindications for the peel, and make sure your client has a clear understanding of the expected outcome.

Facial Devices

Using facial devices such an ultrasonic skin spatula, high frequency, and microcurrent will provide some minor benefits for your client and can be included in any facial series. The effect of electrical facial devices is not long lasting. These treatments will help in a series to get your client's skin to a healthy state.

Dermaplaning may be an option for transgender female clients, but do not dermaplane over vellus hair. Dermaplaning over vellus hair could initiate a reaction that will cause the vellus hair to convert to terminal hair.

Lasers and IPL

Advanced devices, such as lasers, are truly the gold standard for care when it comes hair removal. Make sure you are using a device that is FDA registered for treating your client's skin type. Nd: YAG at 1064 nm is the "color blind," "skin friendly" laser for treating darker skin.

Fractional laser is a terrific option for transgender clients for skin rejuvenation, particularly for issues that transgender female clients want addressed: smaller pores, texture improvements, and fine-line reduction.

Your transgender female clients may be interested in body contouring services to help define a more feminine shape. Radio frequency, cryolipolysis as well as laser lipolysis are all good options to finely sculpt your client's shape into one with a more feminine curve (fig 8.5).

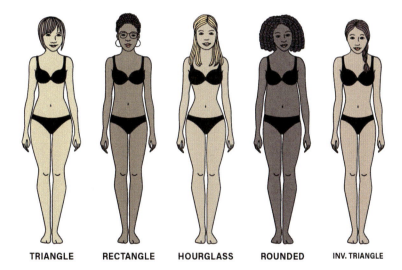

Body contouring can help clients define a more feminine shape. Become familiar with common body shapes to assist in sculpting more feminine curves. Illustration source: mexanichp/Shutterstock.com and Franzi draws/stock.adobe.com, edited by Sarah Jensen.
(8.5)

Combination Treatments

Pretreating your client's skin with a melanocyte-inhibiting product prior to any professional treatment is recommended to avoid the risk of a negative outcome.

You can consider combining treatments in a regimen of facials with advanced devices, chemical peels, and lasers, but your transgender client can achieve a more feminine or masculine look with neuromodulators and dermal fillers integrated in the treatment plan as well.

If injectables are within your scope of practice, it is still my opinion that these types of specialty injections belong in the hands of a medical professional who has expertise in crafting facial contours. A gifted injector can create a stronger jawline for a transgender male client and can round the forehead, enhance the lips, and open the eyes for a transgender female client.

If your client is going to have injections, whether neuromodulators like Botox or dermal fillers, you must time your treatments with the injection schedule. Avoid facial treatments for two weeks after an injection session. Even a chemical peel can cause inflammation and erythema, which can cause the neuromodulator to drift and give your client a lid ptosis.

Home Skincare Recommendations

Depending on your client's transgender journey, you may have to make several home-skincare regimen adjustments. When your client initiates hormonal therapy, the skin is going to have some strong reactions. Transgender women will experience dryness as oil gland production is reduced. Your skin assessment of normal, dry, oily, or sensitive will be important. As the hormone schedule for transgender women is adjusted, your client's skin will undergo reactions and may need home care to support the changes. A skin analysis is recommended at each professional visit to adjust home skin care accordingly.

Your transgender male client may have acne issues due to testosterone and other hormone reactions on the skin. Use the information you already have on treating multi-ethnic skin to build a home care plan using effective products that help reduce keratinization build-up and control *p. acnes* bacteria.

SPF protection is always the correct option for your clients including your transgender clients. Make sure your clients are using makeup foundation or moisturizers with an SPF of 30 or higher.

Conclusion

Part of the satisfaction that comes with this profession is helping your clients feel confident in their own skin. Transgender, multi-ethnic clients have unique challenges concerning skincare. By being knowledgeable, you'll be able to treat transgender clients with confidence and help them build self-esteem.

NOTES

1. "Transgender People, Gender Identity and Gender Expression," American Psychological Association, accessed March 28, 2019, https://www.apa.org/topics/lgbt/transgender.

2. Mere Abrams, "Is There a Difference Between Being Transgender and Transsexual," Healthline, November 21, 2019, https://www.healthline.com/health/transgender/difference-between-transgender-and-transsexual.

3. "Glossary of Terms - Transgender," GLAAD, accessed September 7, 2020, https://www.glaad.org/reference/transgender.

4. B.A. Ginsberg, "Dermatologic Care of the Transgender Patient," *International Journal of Women's Dermatology* 3, no. 1 (March 2017): 65-67, https://doi.org/10.1016/j.ijwd.2016.11.007.

5. "Differences between Male and Female Skin," HL Skin Care, accessed March 28, 2019, https://www.hl-labs.com/pro-info/differences-between-male-and-female-skin.html.

6. Gene de Haan et al., "Non-Prescribed Hormone Use and Barriers to Care for Transgender Women in San Francisco," *LGBT Health* 2, no. 4 (December 2015): 313-23, https://doi.org/10.1089/lgbt.2014.0128.

7. S.N. Mundluru and A.R. Larson, "Medical Dermatologic Conditions in Transgender Women," *International Journal of Women's Dermatology* 4, no. 4 (December 2018): 212-215, https://doi.org/10.1016/j.ijwd.2018.08.008.

8. Mundluru and Larson, "Medical Dermatologic Conditions in Transgender Women," 212-215.

9. "Transgender People and HIV: What We Know," Human Rights Campaign, accessed September 7, 2020, https://www.hrc.org/resources/transgender-people-and-hiv-what-we-know.

10. Ian CT TSE, "Dermatologic Manifestations in HIV Disease," Virtual AIDS Office of Hong Kong, accessed August 17, 2020, https://www.aids.gov.hk/pdf/g190htm/21.htm.

11. Hüsamettin Top and Serkan Balta, "Transsexual Mastectomy: Selection of Appropriate Technique According to Breast Characteristics," *Balkan Medical Journal* 34, no. 2 (March 2017): 147-155, https://doi.org/10.4274/balkanmedj.2016.0093.

Fig 8.2. Landyn Pan, *Gender Pronouns*, infographic, TSER, accessed April 17, 2019, http://www.transstudent.org/pronouns101/.

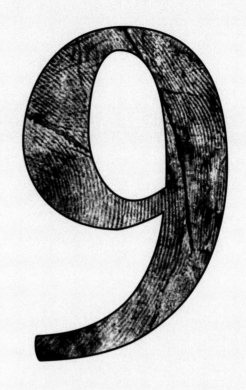

9

CULTURAL APPROPRIATION

CULTURAL APPROPRIATION

Appropriation generally refers to taking something without permission. For instance, congress may vote to appropriate taxes without the public's approval, or a child at the playground may appropriate another child's toy.

The United States borrows or incorporates different cultures on many levels (fig 9.1). Cultural exchange is healthy because it is conducted with appreciation and a sense of equality. Probably the most common cultural exchange is adopting food or meals into our diets from a heritage that is different from our own, such as Mexican or Italian food. We appropriate clothing and jewelry from other cultures as well. Turquoise stones in silver settings, alpaca sweaters, and Scottish plaid are examples of items that many Americans wear but have originated in another culture or country and may not be native to their ancestry.

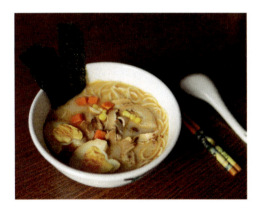

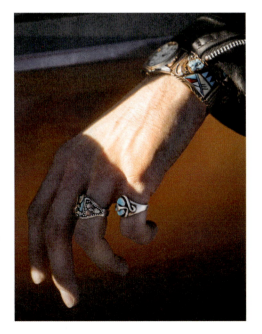

In modern society cultural exchange is common, everything from food to clothing and jewelry may have origins in other cultures. It is important to reflect on the cultural exchanges present in your daily life to make sure they promote appreciation instead of exploitation. Photo Source: (left) Max Oh on Unsplash, (right) Jakob Owens on Unsplash.

(9.1)

Negative cultural appropriation happens when the culture is mocked or adopted without the proper respect (fig 9.2). Wearing a costume that perpetuates negative stereotypes is an example of racist cultural appropriation. Dressing as an Indigenous person, a geisha, or in blackface trivializes the trauma experienced by minorities who have been marginalized, ignored, or oppressed for years.

The Victoria's Secret runway show displayed gross insensitivity when it featured a white model in lingerie wearing an Indigenous headdress in 2017. In Indigenous culture, a headdress is an item worn for sacred events and had to be earned by the wearer. Victoria's Secret's blatant insensitivity demonstrated a lack of respect for Indigenous people.

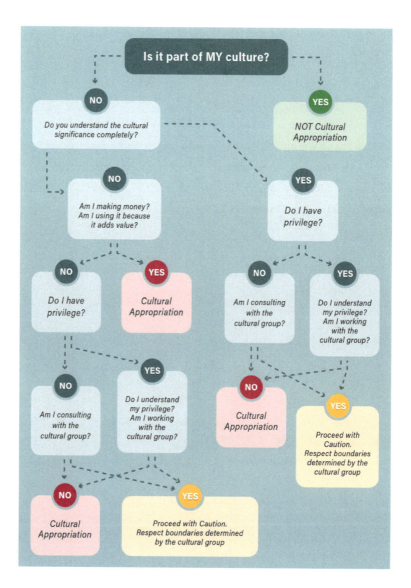

This graphic can help you determine whether the cultural exchange is cultural appreciation or cultural appropriation. Chart Source: Sarah Jensen.

(9.2)

Cultural appropriation is a frequent controversy in the beauty industry. There can be a healthy and collaborative sharing of cultures on one hand, but the adoption of cultural identities must be handled with sensitivity.

Black women have traditional hairstyles including braiding, corn rows, and dreadlocks, and haircare is an important part of Black women's beauty rituals and has been for centuries. White women such as the Kardashians, Katie Perry, and others were celebrated as "edgy" and "urban ethnic" in the news media when they wore their hair in corn rows, which sends the message that Black beauty is only recognized when its style is adopted by the white community, the dominant culture.

The white-dominated beauty industry is often biased against people of color while profiting from their cultural traditions. Ulta Beauty was challenged for its new Frida Kahlo line of cosmetics. It seemed to capitalize on the popularity of Frida Kahlo, but it did not support Mexican heritage and people.

Rihanna quickly acted to remove her highlighter, Geisha Chic, from her Fenty Beauty makeup line once she became aware that it was offensive to Japanese Americans. Geisha means a Japanese girl or woman who is trained to provide entertaining and lighthearted company especially for a man or group of men.[1]

K-beauty is an example of beauty culture appropriation that has been respectfully embraced for the most part. Although recently discovered by Americans, Korean beauty ingredients and rituals have been used for centuries. As US consumers became intrigued and the demand grew, retailers began carrying K-beauty brands while other American brands began producing K-beauty-inspired products.

It seems ironic that people of color continue to face institutionalized racism while some individuals feel threatened by BIPOC while our society endorses white celebrities appropriating other ethnicities' cultures. Having an appreciation for the beauty in other cultures and giving credit and respect to those cultures must happen in the beauty industry in order to promote equality and inclusivity.

Nicki Minaj said, "If you want to enjoy our culture and our lifestyle, then you should also want to know what affects us, what is bothering us, and what we feel is unfair. You shouldn't NOT want to know that."

NOTES

1. Marquaysa Battle, "Rihanna Pulled A Fenty Highlighter That's Offensive To Japanese Culture," Revelist, April 2, 2019, https://www.revelist.com/makeup/rihanna-geisha-chic-cultural-appropriation/15093.

Fig 9.1. Max Oh, *noodle soup on white bowl*, 2019, Photograph, Unsplash, https://unsplash.com/photos/B3VTHOLngWA.

Jakob Owens, *man wearing two gold-colored rings on his left hand*, 2018, Photograph, Unsplash, https://unsplash.com/photos/fG9p2-NXqn4.

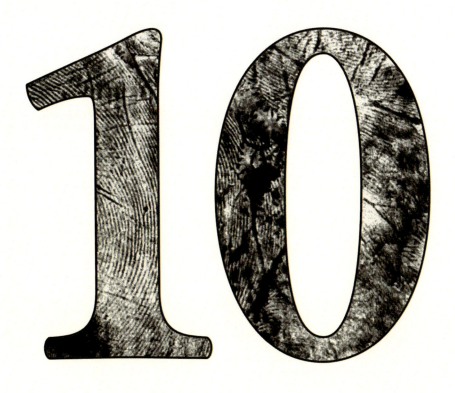

10

SKIN CLASSIFICATION SYSTEMS

SKIN CLASSIFICATION SYSTEMS

Cultures have created skin classification systems for thousands of years. They have been used to create social orders based on wealth, education, political views, skin color, and other factors. For example, the Spanish empire adopted a *casta* system to identify the different races and racial combinations that formed during the colonization of the Americas after 1492. This included Europeans, Indigenous peoples, and slaves from Africa. Paintings described the various combinations (fig 10.1).[1]

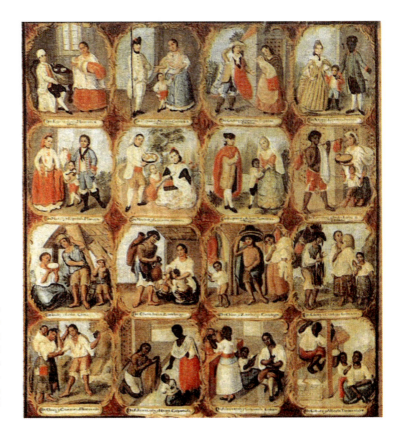

Las castas mexicanas. A caste painting comprised of sixteen scenes that show the dilution of 'pure' blood. Inscriptions near each scene identify the name assigned to the caste. Painting source: Barreda, *Las castas mexicanas,* Real Academia Española.

(10.1)

Felix Von Luschan developed a scale made of thirty-six colored glass tiles that was used for skin classification from the early 1900s until the development of the Fitzpatrick scale in the 1970s (fig 10.2). It was quite subjective since color standardization of the tiles was difficult, and each practitioner may categorize a person's skin color somewhat differently. It had no real medical value but was used in anthropological studies to describe skin color.[2]

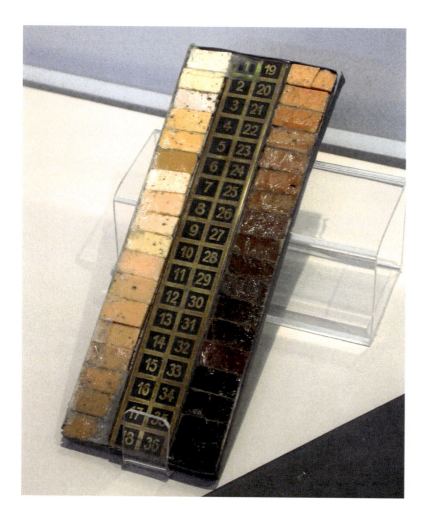

Arranged in a chromatic scale, a set of von Luschan tiles consisted of 36 standardize, opaque glass tiles. Photo source: Ruellan, *Von Luschan's*.
(10.2)

The Fitzpatrick Scale (fig 10.3), considered by many in dermatology as the gold standard in skin classification systems, was created in 1975 by the chairman of Harvard Medical School, Thomas Fitzpatrick. He is considered the father of academic dermatology[3], and his career focus was the study of UV exposure on skin and malignant melanoma. He developed the scale to determine how skin reacts to sun exposure. With the advent of lasers and other advanced devices used in aesthetics, the scale has transitioned into a tool for practitioners who are looking for a predictor of how the skin will react to light energy. The original Fitzpatrick scale did not take ethnic heritage and the skin's response to injury and inflammation into consideration, so it is not always an accurate resource when performing advanced aesthetic treatments.

There are other scales for measuring skin activity, and we will discuss three of them in this chapter.

FITZPATRICK TYPE	EYES	HAIR	UNEXPOSED SKIN	HERITAGE HEREDITY	SKIN REACTION IN UV EXPOSURE
1	Blue, Green	Blonde, Red	Very white Almost translucent, Freckles	English, Irish, Scottish, Northern European	Always burns, Peels with burn, Does not tan
2	Blue, Hazel, Brown	Red, Blonde, Brown	Light	Scandinavian, and same as Fitzpatrick 1	Burns easily, Usually peels, Tans minimally
3	Brown	Dark	Fair to Olive	Spanish, Greek, Italian	Tans well, Burns moderately
4	Dark	Dark	Light brown	Mediterranean, Asian, Hispanic	Tans easily, Burns minimally, Experiences immediate pigment response
5	Dark	Dark	Dark brown	South Asian, Hispanic, Indigenous American, Latin America, Black American	Rarely burns, Tans easily and significantly
6	Dark	Dark	Dark brown, Black	Black American, Aboriginal	Rarely/never burns, Tans easily

The Fitzpatrick Scale. Chart source: Sarah Jensen.
(10.3)

GLOGAU CLASSIFICATION	GLOGAU CHARACTERISTICS	TREATMENT OPTIONS
Type 1	Early photo-aging, No wrinkles Age: 20s to 30s Mild pigmentary changes No keratosis Minimal wrinkles	Sunscreen, Education, Topical tretinoin, Skincare products, Superficial chemical peels, Microdermabrasion, Infused microdermabrasion, Neuromodulators
Type 2	Moderate photo-aging, Wrinkles in motion Age: late 30s or 40s Early sun damage visible Keratosis palpable but not visible Parallel smile lines appearing	Sunscreen, Education, Topical tretinoin, Hyaluronic acid. Skincare products, Medium depth chemical peels, Microdermabrasion, Infused microdermabrasion, Microneedling, Neuromodulators
Type 3	Advanced photo-aging, Wrinkles at rest Age: 50s or older Obvious pigmentation & vascular changes Visible keratosis Skin laxity	Sunscreen, Education, Deep chemical peels, Microneedling, Combination treatments, Laser resurfacing in periorbital and perioral, Skin tightening treatments, Dermal fillers, Neuromodulators
Type 4	Severe photo-aging, Only wrinkles Age: 60s and 70s Yellow-gray skin color & rough texture Prior skin malignancies Wrinkled skin throughout	PDT chemical peel, Microneedling, Full face laser resurfacing, Full face skin tightening, Dermal fillers, Neuromodulators Surgery: Facelift, Browlift, Blepharoplasty

Top Chart
The Glogau Scale with treatment options for Glogau skin types. Chart source: Sarah Jensen. (10.4)

POINTS	CLASSIFICATION
0	Hypopigmentation
I	Minimal and transient hyperpigmentation
II	Minimal and permanent hyperpigmentation
III	Moderate and transient hyperpigmentation
IV	Moderate and permanent hyperpigmentation
V	Severe and permanent hyperpigmentation

Bottom Chart
Hyperpigmentation scale for the Roberts Skin Type Classification. Chart source: Sarah Jensen. (10.5)

Glogau Scale

The Glogau Scale (fig 10.4) was invented in 1996 by Dr. Richard Glogau, a dermatology professor at the University of California San Francisco. It measures the amount of sun damage in white skin.

The Glogau Scale has not been widely adopted, but it is referenced in plastic surgery as a tool for determining appropriateness for surgical facelifts.

Roberts Skin Type Classification

The Roberts Skin Type Classification system was developed by dermatologist Wendy Roberts in 2008. Dr. Roberts' intent was to create a scale that gathered more data points than the Fitzpatrick Scale in order to predict the skin's response to injury and inflammation.[4]

Four factors are evaluated in the Roberts Skin Type Classification:

1. The Fitzpatrick Scale classification

2. The Glogau Scale ranking

3. Hyperpigmentation, specifically the propensity for hyperpigmentation based on the client's natural history for post-inflammatory hyperpigmentation (PIH) (fig 10.5).

4. Skin scarring. Normal skin healing, hypertrophic scarring, and keloid scarring are taken into consideration in this multifaceted skin ranking system.

These four points are combined with a visual and physical examination of the skin as well as test-site reactions. This scale has also not been heavily adopted but offers more comprehensive information to base decisions for skincare treatments.

Baumann Skin Classification

Leslie Baumann, a dermatologist in Florida and professor at the University of Miami, developed the Baumann Skin Classification system in 2004 (fig 10.6). This system evaluates four skin attributes and then categorizes skin into one of sixteen types. Clients complete a questionnaire concerning their skin's reactions and then a skincare professional conducts a physical assessment to confirm some of the answers.

Skin is evaluated as either Oily or Dry, Sensitive or Resistant, Pigmented or Non-Pigmented, and Wrinkle-Prone or Tight. The first letter of each classification is used to describe the skin type. For example, a person may be DSNW, meaning Dry/Sensitive/Non-Pigmented/Wrinkle-Prone.

Dry versus Oily: this category analyzes the amount of sebum the skin produces. Evaluating the stratum corneum for barrier function as well as diet, hormones, stress, and genetics play a huge role in determining this category.

Sensitive versus Resistant: this category analyzes sensitivities to allergens, the presence of inflammation, and the strength of the stratum corneum to protect the skin are the conditions that are evaluated to determine if skin is sensitive or resistant.

Dr. Baumann includes four sub-categories for the Sensitive versus Resistant evaluation:

- Acne: breakouts, whiteheads, and blackheads
- Rosacea: recurrent flushing, redness, and heat sensation in the skin
- Stinging: stinging or burning
- Allergic: redness, itchiness, and flaking

Pigmented versus Non-Pigmented: this category analyzes the skin based on unwanted pigmentation, whether it is melasma, sun-induced lentigines, or PIH. Many pigmentation disorders can be improved with skincare products.

Wrinkle-Prone versus Tight: Genetics play a factor in skin aging and evidence of laxity, but this category includes environmental aging factors. Lifestyle habits such as smoking influence this category.

With the Baumann Skin Classification system, particular categories typically show certain skin conditions. OSNT and OSPT usually experience acne. OSNW and DSNW experience rosacea. This scale does include skin of color differences. Therefore practitioners can feel confident making skincare recommendations based on the Baumann Skin Classification system.

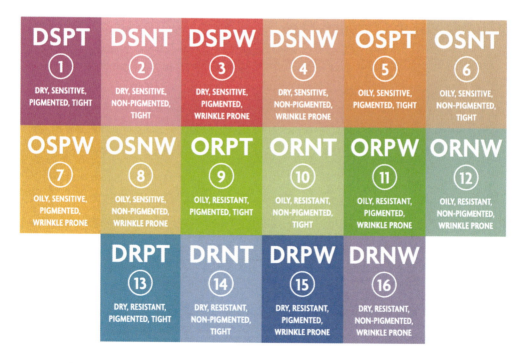

The Baumann Skin Classification system. Graphic source: Sarah Jensen.
(10.6)

Conclusion

The Fitzpatrick scale has been the most widely used scale for skincare professionals to guide selecting appropriate treatments for clients, but it's worth considering alternative systems such as the Roberts Skin Type system or the Baumann Skin Classification system for your practice.

As our country becomes increasingly multi-ethnic and aesthetic treatments grow in popularity, we need to find methods for evaluating our clients' skin in order to offer the safest and most effective treatments. Elevate your profession by being knowledgeable about ethnic and multi-ethnic skin.

NOTES

1. Francisco Herrera, "Theorizing Race in the Americas," Public Books, September 07, 2017, accessed March 28, 2019, https://www.publicbooks.org/theorizing-race-in-the-americas/.

2. Anna K. Swiatoniowski, Ellen E. Quillen, Mark D. Shriver, and Nina G. Jablonski, "Technical Note: Comparing Von Luschan Skin Color Tiles and Modern Spectrophotometry for Measuring Human Skin Pigmentation," *American Journal of Physical Anthropology* 151, no. 2 (June 2013): 325-30. https://doi.org/10.1002/ajpa.22274.

3. "The Fitzpatrick Scale," Derma Health Institute, November 2, 2017, accessed March 28, 2019, https://dermahealthinstitute.com/blog/the-fitzpatrick-scale/.

4. "Roberts Skin Type Classification System : Key to Better Skin Care," Wendy Roberts, MD, accessed March 28, 2019, https://wendyrobertsmd.com/roberts-skin-type-classification-system-key-to-better-skin-care/.

Fig 10.1. Ignacio María Barreda, *Las castas mexicanas*, 1777, oil on canvas, 30.3 x 19.2" (77 x 49 cm), Real Academia Española, Madrid, Spain.

Fig 10.2. Gabriela Ruellan, *Von Luschan's chromatic scale*, January 24, 2016, photograph, Wikipedia, https://commons.wikimedia.org/wiki/File:Von_Luschan%27s_chromatic_scale.jpg.
https://creativecommons.org/licenses/by/3.0/legalcode

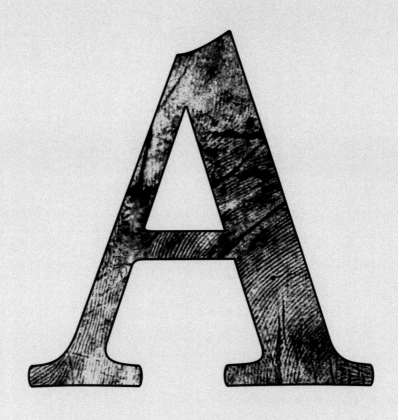

Common Forms

Client Information and Health History

In order to provide you with the most appropriate treatment, we need you to complete the following questionnaire. All information is confidential.

Client Name: _____ Date of Birth: _____

Email Address: _____ Phone Number: _____

Home Address: _____

How were you referred to us? _____ Occupation: _____

Which of the following best describes your skin type? (Please circle one number)

- I. Fair-always burns, never tans
- II. Light skin tones-can burn, sometimes tans
- III. Medium to olive skin tones, tans easily
- IV. Medium to dark skin tones
- V. Brown, moderately pigmented skin
- VI. Black skin

Medical History

Are you currently under the care of a medical professional for any reason? ☐ Yes ☐ No

If yes, for what _____

SEX	☐ Male	☐ Female	☐ Non-binary	Preferred Pronoun?	
HISTORY		YES	NO	DATE/LIST/COMMENTS	
LIST ALL MEDICATIONS, SUPPLEMENTS AND/OR VITAMINS					
Accutane					
Antibiotics					
Birth Control Pills					
Hormones					
Aspirin, Ibuprofen use					
Retin A, Tretinoin					
Metro Gel, Metro Cream					
Antidepressants					
LIST ALLERGIES					
Sun Reactions					
Medication Allergies					
Food Allergies					
Aspirin Allergy					
Latex Allergy					
Lidocaine Allergy					
Hydrocortisone Allergy					
Hydroquinone Allergy					
Other Allergies?					

HISTORY	YES	NO	DATE/LIST/COMMENTS
Diabetes			
Smoking History			
Cold Sores, Herpes			
Bleeding Disorders			
Autoimmune, HIV			
Pregnant, Planning to be			
Pacemaker			
Implants of any kind - dental, breast			
Migraine Headaches			
Glaucoma			
Cancer			
Arthritis			
Hepatitis			
Thyroid Imbalance			
Seizure Disorder			
Active Infection			
Radiation in last 3 months			
SKIN CONDITIONS			
Acne			
Melasma			
Tattoos, Perm. Makeup, Microblading			
Vitiligo			
Keloid Scarring			
Skin/Laser Treatments at another office			If so, when? Results
Botox			If so, when? Results
Fillers			If so, when? Results
Hair Removal			If so, when? Results
Chemical Peels			If so, when? Results
Sun exposure/tanning bed in last week? Self Tanner?			If so, when? Results
HOME SKIN CARE			

☐ I have not experienced a cough, fever or shortness of breath in the last 14 days

☐ I have not tested positive for COVID 19 in the past 14 days

☐ I have not been exposed to someone who has tested positive for COVID 19 in the past 14 days

I understand that, because esthetics involves maintained touch and close physical proximity over an extended period of time, there may be an elevated risk of disease transmission, including COVID-19. By signing this form, I acknowledge that I am aware of the risks involved from receiving treatment at this time, I voluntarily agree to assume those risks, and I release and hold harmless the practitioner from any claims related thereto. I give my consent to receive treatment from this practitioner. I certify that the preceding medical, personal and skin history statements are true and correct. I am aware that it is my responsibility to inform the technician of my current medical and health conditions and to update this information at subsequent visits. A current history is essential for the provider to execute appropriate treatment procedures. I have signed the consent form for this procedure. I have had the opportunity to ask questions prior to the treatment. I accept arbitration as a means of resolution for practice liability.

_____   _____
Signature Client   *Date*

Consultation

Name: _____ Date: _____

Chief Areas of Concern:

Photos? ☐ Yes   ☐ No

Fitz   1   2   3   4   5   6

Skin Type: ☐ Dry ☐ Normal ☐ Sensitive ☐ Combo ☐ Oily ☐ Acneic *Grade Acne* _____

Facial Zone: Conditions:

_____ Dehydrated   _____ Redness

_____ Telangiectasia   _____ Hyperpigmentation

_____ Aging   _____ Fine Lines

_____ Comedones   _____ Sun Damage/Browns

_____ Pustules/Papules   _____ Milia

_____ Cysts   _____ Hyper-Keratinization

_____ Poor Elasticity   _____ Moles

_____ Rosacea   _____ Scarring

_____ Poor Elasticity   _____ Other: _____

Medical History reviewed for contraindications?   ☐ Yes   ☐ No

If yes, list here:

SCORE		0	1	2	3	4
	What is the natural color of client's hair?	Sandy red	Blond	Chestnut, Dark blond	Dark brown	Black
	What is client's eye color?	Light blue, Gray, Green	Blue, Gray, Green	Blue	Dark brown	Brownish black
	What is the color of client's skin that is not exposed to the sun?	Reddish	Very pale	Pale with beige tint	Light brown	Dark brown
	How many freckles on client's unexposed skin areas?	Many	Several	Few	Incidental	None
	What happens when client in the sun TOO long without sunblock?	Painful redness, blistering, peeling	Blistering followed by peeling	Burns, sometimes followed by peeling	Rarely burns	Never had a problem
	How well does client's skin turn brown?	Hardly or not at all	Light color tan	Reasonable tan	Tan very easily	Turn dark very quickly
	Does client turn brown within one day of sun exposure?	Never	Seldom	Sometimes	Often	Always
	How does client's face respond to the sun?	Very sensitive	Sensitive	Normal	Very resistant	Never had a problem
	When was client last exposed to sun or artificial sun treatments?	More than 3 months ago	2-3 months ago	1-2 months ago	Less than 1 month ago	less than 2 weeks ago
	Does client expose area to be treated to sun?	Never	Hardly ever	Sometimes	Often	Always
	TOTAL	What ethnicities does the client identify with?				

00-07 POINTS = SKIN TYPE I **08-16 POINTS = SKIN TYPE II** **17-25 POINTS = SKIN TYPE III**
25-30 POINTS = SKIN TYPE IV **30-40 POINTS = SKIN TYPE V & VI**

Is client preparing for an event?	
Lifestyle	
Diet	
Water intake	
Skincare currently using	

PLAN	# OF SESSIONS	NOTES
Nano-Facial		
Dermaplaning		
Chemical Peel		
OxyGeneo		
Facial Genie		
Nano-Facial		

EXPLANATION	YES	NO
Benefits of Treatment Discussed		
Contraindications Reviewed		
Risk Reviewed: Pigment changes, Swelling, Infection, Scarring, Blistering, Hyper/Hypopigmentation		
Probability of Success Reviewed		
Educated on anticipated consequences if treatment is not performed & alternative treatments available		

☐ Home skin care recommendations:

Reviewed by Skincare Professional   Date

Facial Treatment

Name: _____   Date: _____

Fitz   1   2   3   4   5   6

Skin Type: ☐ Dry ☐ Normal ☐ Sensitive ☐ Combo ☐ Oily ☐ Acneic *Grade Acne* _____

Facial Zone: Conditions:

_____ Dehydrated   _____ Redness
_____ Telangiectasia   _____ Hyperpigmentation
_____ Aging   _____ Fine Lines
_____ Comedones   _____ Sun Damage/Browns
_____ Pustules/Papules   _____ Milia
_____ Cysts   _____ Hyper-keratinization
_____ Poor Elasticity   _____ Moles
_____ Rosacea   _____ Scarring
_____ Poor Elasticity   _____ Other: _____

Treatment _____   Treatment # _____

☐ Goggles *if appropriate*

Treatment Protocol:

☐ Post treatment skin care applied ☐ Yes   ☐ No

☐ Post treatment instructions   ☐ Verbal ☐ Written

☐ Home skin care recommendations

☐ Consult: Intake
☐ Consent Signed
☐ Face Cleansed
   x2 if chemical peel
☐ Photos Taken at EVERY session
☐ Skin Analysis

ZONE 1
ZONE 2
ZONE 3

_____   _____
Reviewed by Skincare Professional   Date

Chemical Peel Protocol

Definition and Purpose: Using a chemical as a substance to create a controlled injury to the upper layers of the skin to improve appearance by refining fine lines, lightening pigmentation, reducing bacteria that cause acneic breakouts and exfoliating dead skin cells. In some instances a wound response is initiated and the stimulation of fibroblasts causes an increase in collagen production, giving the skin a firmer, plumper appearance.

1. Have a 10 cc syringe of water or normal saline available in addition to the peel supplies to flush the client's eyes in the event that peel solution seeps into the eyes.
2. Consult with the client on problem areas.
3. Perform a detailed skin analysis.
4. The client signs the consent form acknowledging the risks and benefits for treatment.
5. Client should be lying on facial bed with hair secured back.
6. Perform a double cleanse on client's skin so it's free from dirt, makeup and oil.
7. Pretreatment photos should be taken to document progress.
8. Prep the skin by wiping with a degreasing solution of alcohol or acetone or prep solution recommended by manufacturer.
9. Apply a medical barrier cream to the creases in the eyes, corners of the mouth and around the nose for extra protection.
10. Prepare neutralizing solution for application after the peel has been applied.
11. Cover the client's eyes with light goggles or 2 x 2 gauze.
12. Pour the peel solution into a medicine cup.
13. Apply the peel with a 2x2 gauze, beginning at the outer perimeter of the face, moving inward toward the nose and center of the face. Reapply to areas that require additional treatment, based on the consultation. Apply additional layers based on manufacturer's recommendations and client's tolerance level. Client should not be at a discomfort level above a 5 on a scale of 0-10.
14. Time peel application according to manufacturer's guidelines. If frosting occurs, apply neutralizer to avoid deeper penetration and potential for hyperpigmentation or hypopigmentation.

15. Client will experience initial warmth that will dissipate as the solution penetrates.

16. After 3-5 minutes, use 4 x 4 cotton pads moistened with ice cold or very cold water and thoroughly rinse skin. During this dilution step, skin may heat up again, but will calm quickly as you rinse. Continue applying cold until client's comfort level is at a 0-1 on a scale of 0-10.

17. Use cooling fan for client comfort with caution as it may cause some self-neutralizing peels to neutralize too quickly with the drying action of the fan.

18. Neutralize peel with recommended solution.

19. Apply post-peel medical barrier cream or other post-treatment skin care.

20. Send client home with verbal and written post-treatment instructions.

21. Document procedure in client record.

Dermaplaning Protocol

Definition and Purpose: To exfoliate the skin and remove superfluous hair.

1. Consult with the client on problem areas.
2. Perform a detailed skin analysis.
3. The client signs the consent form acknowledging the risks and benefits for treatment.
4. Pretreatment photos taken to document progress and condition of skin.
5. Client should be lying on facial bed with hair secured back.
6. Cleanse the face to remove dirt and debris and remove makeup. Rinse well and pat dry with a towel.
7. Use alcohol to sanitize the skin.
8. Apply a light oil based serum. CBD serum works well due to its anti-inflammatory properties.
9. Holding the skin taut between your fingers, keep the blade at a 45 degree angle, use short strokes to sweep the blade on the skin, pulling toward you. You should see tiny bits of dead skin cells lift off the skin. Wipe the accumulating debris on a 4 x 4 gauze.
10. Complete this process on the entire face.
11. Cleanse the face.
12. Apply antioxidant or growth factor serum.
13. Apply moisturizer and SPF.
14. Give client written home care instructions.
15. Document treatment in client record.

Facial Genie Protocol

Definition and Purpose: To cleanse, exfoliate, nourish and protect the skin.

1. Consult with the client on problem areas.
2. Perform a detailed skin analysis.
3. The client signs the consent form acknowledging the risks and benefits for treatment.
4. Pretreatment photos taken to document progress and condition of skin.
5. Client should be lying on facial bed with hair secured back.
6. Apply a woven 4 x 4 gauze to the Facial Genie and secure it with the clear attachment.
7. Dampen the skin. Press the button once. Cleanse the skin with the cleanser of choice, using the gauze as a means of additional exfoliation. The gentle heat and vibration will soften sebum on the face, emulsifying dirt and debris and break up dead skin cells.
8. Rinse well and apply toner.
9. Apply serum of choice and use the Facial Genie LED light for 8 to 10 minutes, with the appropriate LED light wavelength (415 nm-Blue, 535 nm-Green, 620 nm-Red). Ultrasonic vibrations and gentle warmth will assist with circulation and penetration.
10. Do not overstimulate with massage.
11. The serum should be dry enough that it is absorbed by the skin. If not absorbed, use a hot towel to remove excess.
12. Apply an appropriate mask based on your initial skin analysis.
13. Remove mask with warm steamed towel.
14. Apply moisturizer. Use the Facial Genie 620 nm LED Red Light for an additional five minutes for healing and anti-inflammatory purposes.
15. Apply SPF.
16. Send client home with post-treatment instructions.
17. Document treatment in client record.

Facial can be performed with or without steam. In general, it will take about 45 minutes to complete the Facial Genie Treatment.

LED Light Therapy Protocol

Definition and Purpose: Soothe, reduce inflammation, promote healing to the skin.

1. Consult with the client on problem areas.
2. Perform a detailed skin analysis.
3. The client signs the consent form acknowledging the risks and benefits for treatment.
4. Pretreatment photos taken to document progress and condition of skin.
5. Client should be lying on facial bed with hair secured back.
6. The light must be applied to clean bare skin.
7. Apply eye protection.
8. With a hand held device, the face of the device may rest directly on the skin. With a larger LED light unit, apply as close as possible.
9. Time for 10 to 30 minutes, depending on time available for treatment.
10. Remove light.
11. Apply appropriate serum, moisturizer and SPF.
12. Give client written home care instructions.
13. Document treatment in client record.

Nano Facial Protocol

Definition and Purpose: Using nano-chip technology to induce growth of collagen and reduce fine lines, pore size, improve skin texture creating healthy, vibrant skin.

1. Consult with the client on problem areas.
2. Perform a detailed skin analysis.
3. The client signs the consent form acknowledging the risks and benefits for treatment.
4. Pretreatment photos taken to document progress and condition of skin.
5. Client should be lying on facial bed with hair secured back.
6. Apply the nano-chip to the handpiece. Adjust the depth of the nano-chip so it is even with the circular rim of the cartridge. This may be 0.5 mm.
7. Cleanse the face to remove dirt and debris and remove makeup. Rinse well and pat dry with a towel.
8. Disinfect the skin with an alcohol wipe.
9. Divide the face into segments, treating each segment individually.
10. Apply a thin layer of hyaluronic acid to area being treated.
11. Beginning at cheek, do a pass using circular motions across holding the skin taut.
12. Perform a second pass in a diagonal direction.
13. Perform a third pass in a horizontal or vertical direction.

AREA ON FACE BEING TREATED	DEPTH OF TIP
Forehead	0.25 - 0.5 mm
Cheeks	0.5 - 1.0 mm
Upper Lip	0.25 mm
Chin	0.5 - 1.0 mm
Acne Scars	1.0 - 2.0 mm

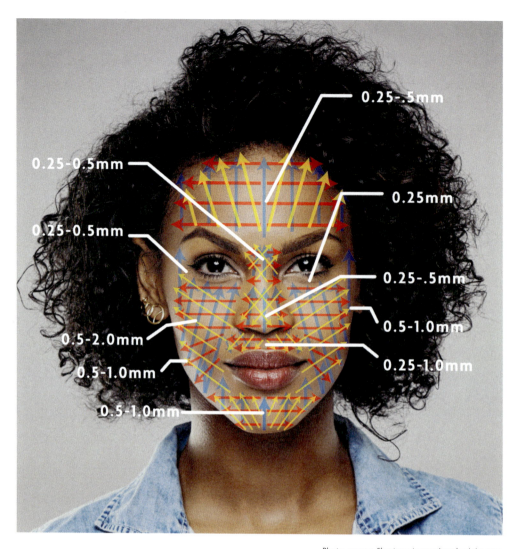

Photo source: Flamingo Images/stock.adobe.com, edited by: Sarah Jensen.

14. Repeat steps 11 through 13 on subsequent sections of the face.

15. Rub in any excess hyaluronic acid serum into the skin.

16. Apply a sheet mask and cool with a jade roller for 5 minutes.

17. Apply SPF

18. Give client written post-treatment instructions.

19. Document the treatment in the client record.

Oxygeneo Protocol

Definition and Purpose: To cleanse, exfoliate, infuse and oxygenate the skin with ultrasound.

1. Consult with the client on problem areas.
2. Perform a detailed skin analysis.
3. Client signs the consent form acknowledging the risks and benefits for treatment.
4. Pretreatment photos taken to document progress and condition of skin.
5. Client should be lying on facial bed with hair secured back.
6. Cleanse the face to remove dirt and debris and remove makeup. Rinse well and pat dry with a towel.
7. Dispense ½ of the packet of Neo Revive gel into a small bowl, reserving the remainder for the ultrasound and massage portion of the treatment.
8. Apply the gel to the face with a facial brush.
9. Attach the Capsugen pod to the OxyGeneo applicator. Adjust the intensity to 7 and the timer to 10 minutes.
10. Glide the Capsugen through the gel very slowly across the entire face. Adjust the intensity according to the client's comfort.
11. Discard the Capsugen pod.
12. Using a tongue blade, remove the excess gel.
13. Cleanse the face again to ensure all Capsugen granules are removed.
14. Apply an antioxidant or growth factor serum to the face, if desired.
15. Using a brush, apply the remaining NeoRevive gel to the face, over the serum.
16. Adjust the intensity to 7 and the timer to 5 minutes.
17. Keeping the ultrasound applicator in contact with the gel, turn on the ultrasound handpiece. The handpiece must remain in contact with the gel at all times, glide the applicator through the gel slowly, covering the entire face, using upward, lifting motions. Avoid the lips. Do not treat beyond the orbital rim. Adjust the intensity according to the client's comfort level.
18. Remove the excess gel with a tongue blade.
19. Rinse the face well with warm water.
20. Apply appropriate moisturizer and SPF.
21. Send client home with written post care instructions.
22. Document treatment in client record.

Chemical Peel Post-Treatment Instructions

DAY ONE: Tight dry; Mild to moderate swelling & redness. Apply post peel cream, keep moist.

DAY TWO: Tight, dry; Mild to moderate swelling & redness. Apply post peel cream, keep moist.

DAY THREE: Skin MAY begin to peel but it's ok if it does not peel. Apply post peel cream and keep moist.

DAY FOUR: Heaviest peeling

DAY FIVE: Most peeling subsiding, but may continue for a couple more days, around hairline mostly. Apply post peel cream and keep moist.

If you have any questions or concerns about any treatment, please contact us at this number: _____

Facial Genie Post-Treatment Instructions

Avoid sun exposure and use a broad spectrum (UVA/UVB) sunscreen to prevent further sun damage.

Avoid skin irritants a few days post-treatment.

If you have any questions or concerns about any treatment, please contact us at this number: _____

LED Light Therapy Post-Treatment Instructions

Avoid sun exposure and use a broad spectrum (UVA/UVB) sunscreen to prevent further sun damage.

If you have any questions or concerns about any treatment, please contact us at this number: _____

Nano Facial Post-Treatment Instructions

Avoid sun exposure and use a broad spectrum (UVA/UVB) sunscreen to prevent further sun damage

Avoid skin irritants a few days post-treatment.

If you have any questions or concerns about any treatment, please contact us at this number: _____

Oxygeneo Facial Post-Treatment Instructions

Avoid sun exposure and use a broad spectrum (UVA/UVB) sunscreen to prevent further sun damage.

Avoid skin irritants a few days post-treatment.

If you have any questions or concerns about any treatment, please contact us at this number: _____

Dermaplaning Post-Treatment Instructions

Avoid sun exposure and use a broad spectrum (UVA/UVB) sunscreen to prevent further sun damage.

Avoid skin irritants a few days post-treatment.

If you have any questions or concerns about any treatment, please contact us at this number: _____

Consent for Chemical Peel

Client Name: _____

You have a right to be informed about your skin and its treatment, so that you may decide whether or not to undergo this procedure after knowing the risks and hazards involved. This disclosure is not meant to scare or alarm you. It is an effort to make you better informed so you may give or withhold your consent for treatment.

I voluntarily request that _____ perform the chemical peel procedure. I acknowledge that I have been informed that this cosmetic procedure is intended to remove surface layers of the skin to improve the vitality of the skin.

Medical strength peels, despite their high levels of efficacy and safety, are not free of side effects. Erythema (redness) and edema (swelling) of the treated area can occur but usually subsides within a few hours but can last up to seven days or longer. Irritation, itching and/or mild burning sensation or pain similar to sunburn may occur within 48 hours of treatment.

Pigmentary changes such as hyperpigmentation or hypopigmenation of the skin in the treated areas can occasionally occur. Mostly it is transient, lasting up to 6 months, but in rare cases it can be permanent. These pigmentary changes may occur despite appropriate protection from the sun so it is important to use sunscreen of SPF 25 or higher when exposed to the sun.

I understand that complications can include whiteheads, cold sores, infection, scarring, numbness and permanent discoloration, particularly in people with darker colored skin.

No guarantee, warranty, or assurance has been made to me as to the results that may be obtained. I am aware that follow-up may be necessary to achieve desired results. Most clients require a number of treatments over several months with gradual results occurring over this time period. Clinical results will vary per individual. I agree to all safety precautions and regulations during the treatment. No refunds are possible for treatments received.

I have received a copy of the Post-Treatment Instructions. I agree to follow these instructions carefully. I understand that compliance with recommended pre and post procedures guidelines are crucial for healing, prevention of scarring, and other side effects and complications such as hyperpigmentation, hypopigmentation and other skin textural changes.

ACKNOWLEDGMENT

I understand and acknowledge that payments for the above procedure are non-refundable. Unused prepaid treatments may be exchanged for credit only.

By my signature below, I certify that I have read and fully understand this agreement. All of my questions have been answered to my satisfaction and I consent to the terms of this agreement. Alternative methods of treatment and their risks and benefits have been explained to me and I understand I have the right to refuse treatment. I release the clinic, its technicians, and staff from liability associated with this procedure. This consent form is freely and voluntarily executed and binding upon my spouse, relatives, legal representatives, heirs, administrators, successors and assigns. I consent to before and after photos for comparison.

_____   _____
Signature Client   *Date*

Consent for Dermaplaning

Client Name: _____

You have a right to be informed about your skin and its treatment, so that you may decide whether or not to undergo this procedure after knowing the risks and hazards involved. This disclosure is not meant to scare or alarm you. It is an effort to make you better informed so you may give or withhold your consent for treatment.

I voluntarily request that _____ perform the dermaplaning procedure. I acknowledge that I have been informed that this cosmetic procedure is intended to exfoliate the skin to improve the vitality of the skin and remove superfluous hair.

Dermaplaning, despite its high levels of efficacy and safety, is not free of side effects. Erythema (redness) and edema (swelling) of the treated area can occur but usually subsides within a few hours but can last up to seven days or longer. Irritation, itching and/or mild burning sensation or pain similar to sunburn may occur within 48 hours of treatment.

Pigmentary changes such as hyperpigmentation or hypopigmenation of the skin in the treated areas may rarely occur if a skin abrasion occurs during the treatment. Mostly it is transient, lasting up to 6 months, but in rare cases it can be permanent. These pigmentary changes may occur despite appropriate protection from the sun so it is important to use sunscreen of SPF 25 or higher when exposed to the sun.

I understand that complications can include whiteheads, cold sores, infection, scarring, numbness and permanent discoloration, particularly in people with darker colored skin.

No guarantee, warranty, or assurance has been made to me as to the results that may be obtained. I am aware that follow-up may be necessary to achieve desired results. Clinical results will vary per individual. I agree to all safety precautions and regulations during the treatment. No refunds are possible for treatments received.

I have received a copy of the Post-Treatment Instructions. I agree to follow these instructions carefully. I understand that compliance with recommended pre and post procedures guidelines are crucial for healing, prevention of scarring, and other side effects and complications such as hyperpigmentation, hypopigmentation and other skin textural changes.

ACKNOWLEDGMENT

I understand and acknowledge that payments for the above procedure are non-refundable. Unused prepaid treatments may be exchanged for credit only.

By my signature below, I certify that I have read and fully understand this agreement. All of my questions have been answered to my satisfaction and I consent to the terms of this agreement. Alternative methods of treatment and their risks and benefits have been explained to me and I understand I have the right to refuse treatment. I release the clinic, its technicians, and staff from liability associated with this procedure. This consent form is freely and voluntarily executed and binding upon my spouse, relatives, legal representatives, heirs, administrators, successors and assigns. I consent to before and after photos for comparison.

_____   _____
Signature Client   *Date*

Consent for Facial Genie

Client Name: _____

You have a right to be informed about your skin and its treatment, so that you may decide whether or not to undergo this procedure after knowing the risks and hazards involved. This disclosure is not meant to scare or alarm you. It is an effort to make you better informed so you may give or withhold your consent for treatment.

I voluntarily request that _____ perform a facial using the Facial Genie. I acknowledge that I have been informed that this cosmetic procedure is intended to cleanse and hydrate the skin to improve the vitality of the skin.

Facial Genie, despite its high level of efficacy and safety, is not free of side effects. Erythema (redness) and edema (swelling) of the treated area can occur but usually subsides within a few hours but can last up to seven days or longer. Irritation, itching and/or mild burning sensation or pain similar to sunburn may occur within 48 hours of treatment.

No guarantee, warranty, or assurance has been made to me as to the results that may be obtained. I am aware that follow-up may be necessary to achieve desired results. Most clients require a number of treatments over several months with gradual results occurring over this time period. Clinical results will vary per individual. I agree to all safety precautions and regulations during the treatment. No refunds are possible for treatments received.

I have received a copy of the Post-Treatment Instructions. I agree to follow these instructions carefully. I understand that compliance with recommended pre and post procedures guidelines are crucial for healing.

ACKNOWLEDGMENT

I understand and acknowledge that payments for the above procedure are non-refundable. Unused prepaid treatments may be exchanged for credit only.

By my signature below, I certify that I have read and fully understand this agreement. All of my questions have been answered to my satisfaction and I consent to the terms of this agreement. Alternative methods of treatment and their risks and benefits have been explained to me and I understand I have the right to refuse treatment. I release the clinic, its technicians, and staff from liability associated with this procedure. This consent form is freely and voluntarily executed and binding upon my spouse, relatives, legal representatives, heirs, administrators, successors and assigns. I consent to before and after photos for comparison.

_____   _____
Signature Client   *Date*

Consent for LED Light Therapy

Client Name: _____

You have a right to be informed about your skin and its treatment, so that you may decide whether or not to undergo this procedure after knowing the risks and hazards involved. This disclosure is not meant to scare or alarm you. It is an effort to make you better informed so you may give or withhold your consent for treatment.

I voluntarily request that _____ perform the LED Light Therapy procedure. I acknowledge that I have been informed that this cosmetic procedure is intended to improve the vitality of the skin.

LED Light Therapy has a high level of efficacy and safety and there are no long lasting reported side effects. Erythema (redness) of the treated area can occur but usually subsides within a few hours..

No guarantee, warranty, or assurance has been made to me as to the results that may be obtained. I am aware that follow-up may be necessary to achieve desired results. Clinical results will vary per individual. I agree to all safety precautions and regulations during the treatment. No refunds are possible for treatments received.

I have received a copy of the Post-Treatment Instructions. I agree to follow these instructions carefully. I understand that compliance with recommended pre and post procedures guidelines are crucial for healing.

ACKNOWLEDGMENT

I understand and acknowledge that payments for the above procedure are non-refundable. Unused prepaid treatments may be exchanged for credit only.

By my signature below, I certify that I have read and fully understand this agreement. All of my questions have been answered to my satisfaction and I consent to the terms of this agreement. Alternative methods of treatment and their risks and benefits have been explained to me and I understand I have the right to refuse treatment. I release the clinic, its technicians, and staff from liability associated with this procedure. This consent form is freely and voluntarily executed and binding upon my spouse, relatives, legal representatives, heirs, administrators, successors and assigns. I consent to before and after photos for comparison.

_____   _____
Signature Client   Date

Consent for Nano Facial

Client Name: _____

You have a right to be informed about your skin and its treatment, so that you may decide whether or not to undergo this procedure after knowing the risks and hazards involved. This disclosure is not meant to scare or alarm you. It is an effort to make you better informed so you may give or withhold your consent for treatment.

I voluntarily request that _____ perform the Nano Facial procedure. I acknowledge that I have been informed that this cosmetic procedure is intended to infuse the skin to improve the vitality of the skin.

The Nano Facial, despite its high levels of efficacy and safety, is not free of side effects. Erythema (redness) and edema (swelling) of the treated area can occur but usually subsides within a few hours but can last up to seven days or longer. Irritation, itching and/or mild burning sensation or pain similar to sunburn may occur within 48 hours of treatment.

Pigmentary changes such as hyperpigmentation or hypopigmenation of the skin in the treated areas may rarely occur. Mostly it is transient, lasting up to 6 months, but in rare cases it can be permanent. These pigmentary changes may occur despite appropriate protection from the sun so it is important to use sunscreen of SPF 25 or higher when exposed to the sun.

I understand that complications can include whiteheads, cold sores, infection, scarring, numbness and permanent discoloration, particularly in people with darker colored skin.

No guarantee, warranty, or assurance has been made to me as to the results that may be obtained. I am aware that follow-up may be necessary to achieve desired results. Most clients require a number of treatments over several months with gradual results occurring over this time period. Clinical results will vary per individual. I agree to all safety precautions and regulations during the treatment. No refunds are possible for treatments received.

I have received a copy of the Post-Treatment Instructions. I agree to follow these instructions carefully. I understand that compliance with recommended pre and post procedures guidelines are crucial for healing, prevention of scarring, and other side effects and complications such as hyperpigmentation, hypopigmentation and other skin textural changes.

ACKNOWLEDGMENT

I understand and acknowledge that payments for the above procedure are non-refundable. Unused prepaid treatments may be exchanged for credit only.

By my signature below, I certify that I have read and fully understand this agreement. All of my questions have been answered to my satisfaction and I consent to the terms of this agreement. Alternative methods of treatment and their risks and benefits have been explained to me and I understand I have the right to refuse treatment. I release the clinic, its technicians, and staff from liability associated with this procedure. This consent form is freely and voluntarily executed and binding upon my spouse, relatives, legal representatives, heirs, administrators, successors and assigns. I consent to before and after photos for comparison.

_____   _____
Signature Client   *Date*

Consent for OxyGeneo

Client Name: _____

You have a right to be informed about your skin and its treatment, so that you may decide whether or not to undergo this procedure after knowing the risks and hazards involved. This disclosure is not meant to scare or alarm you. It is an effort to make you better informed so you may give or withhold your consent for treatment.

I voluntarily request that _____ perform the OxyGeneo procedure. I acknowledge that I have been informed that this cosmetic procedure is intended to exfoliate and oxygenate the skin to improve the vitality of the skin.

OxyGeneo, despite its high level of efficacy and safety, is not free of side effects. Erythema (redness) and edema (swelling) of the treated area can occur but usually subsides within a few hours but can last up to seven days or longer. Irritation, itching and/or mild burning sensation or pain similar to sunburn may occur within 48 hours of treatment.

Pigmentary changes such as hyperpigmentation or hypopigmenation of the skin in the treated areas can occasionally occur. Mostly it is transient, lasting up to 6 months, but in rare cases it can be permanent. These pigmentary changes may occur despite appropriate protection from the sun so it is important to use sunscreen of SPF 25 or higher when exposed to the sun.

I understand that complications can include whiteheads, cold sores, infection, scarring, numbness and permanent discoloration, particularly in people with darker colored skin.

No guarantee, warranty, or assurance has been made to me as to the results that may be obtained. I am aware that follow-up may be necessary to achieve desired results. Most clients require a number of treatments over several months with gradual results occurring over this time period. Clinical results will vary per individual. I agree to all safety precautions and regulations during the treatment. No refunds are possible for treatments received.

I have received a copy of the Post-Treatment Instructions. I agree to follow these instructions carefully. I understand that compliance with recommended pre and post procedures guidelines are crucial for healing, prevention of scarring, and other side effects and complications such as hyperpigmentation, hypopigmentation and other skin textural changes.

ACKNOWLEDGMENT

I understand and acknowledge that payments for the above procedure are non-refundable. Unused prepaid treatments may be exchanged for credit only.

By my signature below, I certify that I have read and fully understand this agreement. All of my questions have been answered to my satisfaction and I consent to the terms of this agreement. Alternative methods of treatment and their risks and benefits have been explained to me and I understand I have the right to refuse treatment. I release the clinic, its technicians, and staff from liability associated with this procedure. This consent form is freely and voluntarily executed and binding upon my spouse, relatives, legal representatives, heirs, administrators, successors and assigns. I consent to before and after photos for comparison.

_____ _____
Signature Client   *Date*

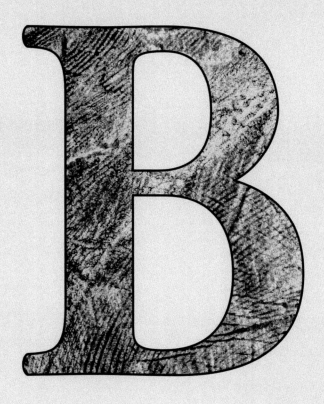

GLOSSARY

A   ANTHROPOLOGY The study of the origins and cultural development, social customs, and beliefs of the human race.

APPROPRIATION The action of taking something for one's own use, typically without the owner's permission.

ATOPIC DERMATITIS Chronic skin inflammation causing itching and redness, often due to skin sensitivity. It may improve for a time but relapse periodically. Skin barrier is compromised, with erythema, inflammation and itchiness.

AUTOIMMUNE DISEASE When the body's infection fighting system attacks healthy cells in the body.

AYURVEDA One of the world's oldest holistic healing systems developed more than 3,000 years ago in India. It is based on the belief that health and wellness depend on a delicate balance between the mind, body, and spirit. Its main goal is to promote good health, not fight disease, but treatments may be geared toward specific health problems.

B   BAUMANN SKIN TYPING SYSTEM A method of guiding practitioners in selecting the most appropriate ingredients for skincare products after evaluating with a scientifically validated questionnaire on skin response. It was developed by Dr. Leslie Baumann in 2004.

BURQA A loose garment worn by Muslim women that covers the entire body with a veiled opening for the eyes.

C   CASTA SYSTEM A classification system designed by the Spanish Empire during the colonization of the Americas to describe the variety of races and racial combinations, including Indigenous, European, and African slaves.

CHITLINS Fried or boiled pig intestines.

COLLAGEN INDUCTION THERAPY A minimally-invasive skin treatment that works to improve fine lines, wrinkles, pore size, and stimulate the production of collagen. Microneedling and fractional resurfacing are both forms of collagen induction therapy. These treatments are popular because they are relatively safe for all skin types and offer predictable good results with little to no social downtime.

COLONIALISM The practice of a country to gain political control over another country, occupying it, and exploiting it for financial gain.

D   DERMATOSIS PAPULOSA NIGRA (DPN) Condition found in Black skin where the cheeks and eye area have dark-brown-to-black pigmented lesions that are non-cancerous.

DIABETES A multifaceted disease that affects the body's ability to process blood sugar. It has systemic symptoms that affect wound healing, nerve function, cardiac function, and more.

DOSHA Three energies that balance every person's life in the Ayurvedic holistic medicine philosophy. The three energies are called Pitta, Vata and Kapha. Each energy has characteristics specific to the five life forces: air, earth, fire, water, and space.

E   EDEMA Swelling due to injury, inflammation, or constriction of lymphatic flow.

ERYTHEMA Abnormal redness in the skin, typically due to inflammation.

F   FIBROIDS Firm, compact tumors that develop in the uterus and are made of smooth muscle cells and fibrous connective tissue.

FITZPATRICK SCALE A numerical classification system for human skin color developed in 1975 by Thomas B. Fitzpatrick as a way to estimate the response of different types of skin to ultraviolet (UV) light.

FTM Abbreviation for a person who is transitioning or has transitioned from female to male. The term is considered contentious by transgender community. The preferred term is transgender man or transgender male client.

G   GENDER NON-CONFORMING A term used to describe some individuals whose gender expression is different from conventional expectations of masculinity and femininity. Please note that not all gender non-conforming people identify as transgender; nor are all transgender people gender non-conforming. Many people have gender expressions that are not entirely conventional – that fact alone does not make them transgender. Many transgender men and women have gender expressions that are conventionally masculine or feminine. Simply being transgender does not make someone gender non-conforming. The term is not a synonym for transgender or transsexual and should only be used if someone self-identifies as gender non-conforming.

GLOGAU SCALE A skin classification system developed by Richard Glogau as a way to measure photo-aging in white/European skin.

GRANULOMA A structure formed during a period of inflammation as the body's immune system attempts to wall off substances that it identifies as foreign but is unable to remove.

H HEMOGLOBIN Protein responsible for transporting oxygen in the blood.

HEMOSIDERIN STAINING A brown discoloration that appears on the skin when broken blood vessels leave residue from the protein that stores iron in the blood.

HIRSUTISM Unwanted male pattern hair growth on a woman, including dark coarse hair on the face.

HYDROPHILIC A strong affinity for water. In reference to chemical peel acids, alpha hydroxyl acids are hydrophilic.

HYDROQUINONE A topical skin-lightening product that inhibits the production of tyrosinase, an enzyme needed for melanin production.

HYPERTROPHIC SCAR An abnormal healing response to a skin injury that causes an overgrowth of skin tissue that exceeds the original scar formation.

I ICHTHYOSIS PREMATURITY SYNDROME A rare genetic disorder almost exclusive to people of Nordic descent. The child is born prematurely and has thick, dry, scaly skin that persists throughout life.

INDIGENOUS Native, originating in the country or area.

K KAPHA The largest of the three ayurvedic body types, with wide hips and shoulders, thick hair, and strong physical stamina. Kapha lends structure, solidity, and cohesiveness to all things, and is therefore associated with the earth and water elements. Kapha also embodies the watery energies of love and compassion. This dosha hydrates all cells and systems, lubricates the joints, moisturizes the skin, maintains immunity, and protects tissues.

KELOID An overgrowth of scar tissue that stays within the original scar formation.

L LIPOPHILIC A strong affinity for oils. In reference to chemical peel acids, salicylic acids are lipophilic.

LUPUS ERYTHEMATOSUS An autoimmune disorder where the body attacks healthy tissue, affecting the skin, joints, kidneys, and brain. Physical symptoms include a butterfly shape pattern rash on the cheeks and nose, fatigue, swollen joints, fever, and edema. It is more common in Black skin and in Asian skin.

M MAST CELLS A large granular cell that is common in skin and connective tissue that produces heparin (blood blotting agent), histamine (causes blood vessels to dilate during inflammation) and serotonin (a chemical that releases positive feelings in the brain).

MEHNDI KI RAAT Applying an elaborate design of henna on the hands of the bride and groom the day before a wedding.

MELANOCYTE Melanin producing cell locating in the basal layer of the epidermis.

MELANOPHAGE A melanin containing macrophage found in pigmented lesions.

MELANOSOME The structure in a melanin producing cell that actually produces the melanin.

MELASMA A hyperpigmentation disorder characterized by bilateral pigmentation commonly found on the cheeks, forehead, upper lip, chin, and jawline, often from hormonal imbalance disorders.

MILLENNIALS A person born from 1981 through 1996.

MONOCHROMATIC A single wavelength or frequency.

MTF Abbreviation for a person who is transitioning or has transitioned from male to female. The term is considered contentious by transgender community. The preferred term is transgender woman or transgender female client.

MULTI-ETHNIC Referring to several ethnic groups, a blending of different ethnicities.

N NEUROMODULATORS Injectable neuromodulators that influence the transmission of nerve impulses in facial muscles to decrease the appearance of fine lines and wrinkles. Botox, Dysport, and Xeomin are the most common neuromodulators in the aesthetic arena.

NORDIC Referring to people who are from Scandinavia, Iceland, Greenland, and Ireland.

O OCHRONOSIS Hyperpigmentation that occurs after excessive application of topical hydroquinone. It is usually a permanent discoloration, even when the hydroquinone application is stopped.

P PARADOXICAL HAIR GROWTH A rare side effect after laser hair removal that causes vellus hair growth in the area that was treated and is most common in South Asian populations.

PERIOCULAR Surrounding the eye.

PHOTOSENSITIZING MEDICATION A medication that causes an inflammatory response in the skin when it comes in contact with light energy.

PITTA One of the three Ayurvedic body types associated with athletic builds, Pitta is closely related to intelligence, understanding as well as the digestion of foods, thoughts, emotions, and experiences. It governs nutrition and metabolism, body temperature, and the light of understanding.

POLYCYSTIC OVARIAN SYNDROME (PCOS) A hormonal condition characterized by irregular menstruation, excess hair growth and obesity, and an increased risk of diabetes.

POST-INFLAMMATORY HYPERPIGMENTATION (PIH) A condition in which an injury or inflammation to the skin causes increased pigment production.

PSEUDOFOLLICULITIS BARBAE Commonly called razor bumps, it occurs in 60% of people with curly hair. Highly curved hairs grow back into the skin causing inflammation in the skin.

PTOSIS Drooping of the upper eyelid.

R ROBERTS SKIN TYPE SYSTEM A classification system that collects the data from the Fitzpatrick scale, the Glogau scale, the way the client hyperpigments, and the client's scarring potential.

S SARCOIDOSIS An inflammatory disease that affects multiple organs in the body, but mostly the lungs and lymph glands. Abnormal masses or nodules (called granulomas) consisting of inflamed tissues form in certain organs of the body.

SHADEISM Discrimination against an individual based not just on their perceived race but on their darker skin tone.

SOUL FOOD A variety of cuisine originating in the Southeastern United States, it is derived from African American culture with Indigenous American influences.

T TRANSEPIDERMAL WATER LOSS (TEWL) Water that passively evaporates through skin to the external environment.

TRANSGENDER An umbrella term for persons whose gender identity and gender expression or behavior does not conform to the sex they were assigned at birth.

TYROSINASE An enzyme that acts as a catalyst with melanocytes to produce pigment.

V VATA A lean and muscular body type in Ayurvedic medicine, quick-thinking and fast-moving. Vata governs all movement in the mind and body. It controls blood flow, elimination of wastes, breathing and the movement of thoughts across the mind. Since Pitta and Kapha cannot move without it, Vata is considered the leader of the three Ayurvedic Principles in the body.

ACKNOWLEDGMENTS

I am fortunate to live in a world where I am connected to many talented people. I'd like to give special thanks to those who helped make this book a reality.

Sarah Jensen is a steady influence on creating inclusivity. Spectrum has been incredibly blessed to have her skills and talents with graphic design as well as her insights into how to better tell the story.

JoElle Lee's decision to come to Portland in July 2018 played a solidifying role in the decision to redefine Spectrum's curriculum. I admire her courage to travel and speak the message about multi-ethnic skin.

Mark Nielsen keeps me grounded and provides unequaled support in any endeavor.

Aliesh Pierce is a thoughtful advocate for equality and an accomplished educator.

Megan Rayo gave me the honest feedback that tipped my thought processes in the direction of ethnicity and the need to become better educated myself. Her commitment to the cause warms my soul.

Jason Thomas is a brilliant editor and fact checker. He took challenging information and created clarity and understanding.

The Spectrum staff are a wonderful team of smart, collaborative people who make coming to work a joy.

Spectrum Students. I am honored to have students choose Spectrum for their esthetic education. I am committed to providing the very best education so they can elevate the industry and enjoy a long and rewarding career in skincare. Their enthusiasm for life is inspiring.

Made in the USA
Columbia, SC
10 October 2020